Unclog YOUR Arteries

First published in Australia in 2008 by

New Holland Publishers (Australia) Pty Ltd

Sydney * Auckland * London * Cape Town

1/66 Gibbes Street Chatswood NSW 2067 Australia

* 218 Lake Road Northcoate Auckland New Zealand

* New Edgeware Road London W2 2EA United Kingdom

* 80 McKenzie Street Cape Town 8001 South Africa

Copyright © 2008 in text: Ian Hamilton-Craig

Copyright © 2008 New Holland Publishers (Australia) Pty Ltd

National Library of Australia Cataloguing in Publication data:

Hamilton-Craig, Ian, 1944–

Unclog your arteries / author, Ian Hamilton-Craig.

ISBN: 9781741106039 (pbk.) :

Includes index.

Arteries--Diseases--Prevention--Diet therapy. Arteries--Diseases--Prevention.

Heart--Diseases--Prevention--Diet therapy. Heart--Diseases--Prevention. Cookery. Health.

616.105

Publisher: Fiona Schultz

Editor: Jenny Scepanovic

Managing Editor: Lliane Clarke

Designer: Natasha Hayles

Illustrations: Brett Fisher

Production Assistant: Liz Malcolm

Printer: McPherson's Printing Group

10 9 8 7 6 5 4 3 2 1

Unclog
YOUR
Arteries

WITHDRAWN

PREVENT HEART ATTACK AND STROKE
AND LIVE A LONGER. HEALTHIER LIFE

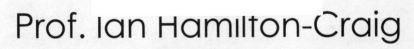

Prof. Ian Hamilton-Craig

NEW
HOLLAND

Dedication

To Marina, for her professional skills and support,
and Christian, who will continue clinical practice and research in
unclogging the arteries.

Foreword

Large numbers of us are living longer, healthier lives due to the enormous advances that have been made in the understanding and treatment of cardiovascular disease. This is a comparatively recent change. Lord Howard Florey (1898–1968), the Adelaide-born scientist who shared the 1945 Nobel Prize for the development of penicillin, was so compromised by anginal pain through the last decade of his life that he had traffic lights on the door of his office. Green meant that it was OK to knock and come in; orange that you would enter at your own risk; and red that you shouldn't even think about it.

Sir Ian Clunies Ross, the charismatic veterinary scientist who led and transformed the CSIRO, died suddenly at age 60 from a heart attack. Both men were sufficiently well regarded that their faces were, at one time or other, displayed on Australian bank notes.

My personal situation is such that I could have expected to share their fate at a fairly early age. A close friend and I tried to resuscitate my 48-year-old father as he died on our lounge-room floor from a second heart attack. We had always thought that his father, a plumber, succumbed to pneumonia after he fell off a roof. Recently, we got hold of his death certificate and found that he was also suffering from cardiovascular disease. With this family history, I had always eaten a low fat diet, exercised and had regular health checks. I first saw a competent cardiologist when, at age 52, I started to develop nocturnal angina. His diagnosis of high blood pressure, high blood cholesterol, and a terrible LDL/HDL ratio undoubtedly saved my life, and meant that I was in good physical shape when I went to Stockholm to receive the 1996 Nobel Prize.

Over the years, I learned that my LDLs are so dense that they would probably drop through any floor I happen to bleed on. I've worked my way up the tree of efficacy for every statin that has been available, and recently added ezetimibe as an additional protection.

Needless to say, I believe very strongly that collaborations between those in academic medicine who often make the basic science discoveries and the chemists, biologists, clinical trial groups and so forth in the private sector drug companies have been enormously productive for humanity.

Unclog Your Arteries represents a continuation of that interaction and is a helpful, clearly written and informative read for any medical professional or intelligent lay reader who has to deal with the blood cholesterol issue.

Professor Peter Doherty
1996 Nobel Laureate for Medicine
1997 Australian of the Year

Contents

Foreword   5
Introduction   10
List of acronyms and common terms   12

Part I: Of Arteries and Coronaries

1: What is Clogging of the Arteries?   16
2: Plaques in the Arteries   23
3: What Causes Clogging?   26
4: Getting Your Arteries Checked Out   31
5: Heart Attack   37
6: Risk Factors for Heart Attack and Stroke   44
7: Measuring Your Risk of Heart Attack and Stroke   50

Part II: All About Blood Fats

8:   Cholesterol, Triglycerides and Lipoproteins   58
9:   Good and Bad Cholesterol   63
10: Blood Fat Levels in Adults and Children   71
11: High Blood Fat Levels—Acquired or Inherited?   77
12: Testing Your Blood Cholesterol Level   88
13: Balancing the Body's Cholesterol   91

Part III: You Are Your Arteries

14:    Food Fat: The Facts   98
15:    Something Fishy   106
16:    Health Supplements   112
17:    The Effects of Alcohol   120
18:    For the Love of Coffee   126
19:    Controlling Those Carbs   130
20:    Flab is Not Fab   135
21:    Blood Glucose Disorders   141
22:    Prohibited and Forbidden: Cigarettes   147
23:    The Fitness Factor   152

Part IV: Coming Clean with Prof Ian

24:    The SAFE Program   162
25:    A Seven Step Plan to Clear Arteries   171
26:    How Low Do You Go?   177
27:    Success Stories from My Casebook   182

Part V: The Magic of Modern Medicine

28:   Medication—Oldies But Goodies   198
29:   Statins: The Magic Bullets   204
30:   The Latest and Greatest Medications   215
31:   Lowering Triglyceride Levels with Drugs   222
32:   Tablets Only Work if You Take Them   229
33:   Surgery and Mechanical Unclogging   237

Part VI: Targeted Groups

34:   Unclogging Women's Arteries   244
35:   Unclogging Children's Arteries   248
36:   Unclogging Arteries in the Elderly   251
37:   Unclogging Arteries after Heart Attack or Surgery   256

Part VII: Low-Chol Cuisine

Changing Old Habits   263
Breakfast   265
Nibbles   269
Vegetable Dishes   272
Soups   276
Main Courses   281
Puddings and Desserts   289

Appendix   292
References   300
Index   301

Introduction

I am a scientist by both training and inclination. I have always enjoyed chemistry, maths, physiology, biology, physics and other such subjects. But my patients have me beaten! For years, I've been treating people who have suffered heart attacks or strokes. No matter how carefully I explain the science and the chemistry of these disorders, I almost inevitably get the same response: 'OK! So my arteries aren't as clear as they ought to be. Can you tell me how to unclog them?' (Sometimes they say 'unblock' or 'clear out' or 'clean out' or even 'un-fuzz', but the most popular term remains 'unclog'.)

The hardening/clogging/fuzzing/blocking of arteries is what leads to heart attack and stroke (cardiovascular disease). My patients want to know what they can do, or what they can take, to help clear their arteries of the dangerous plaque that has built up inside them, like rust inside a water pipe, and has led to complete or partial blockage.

My reply has been: 'There's now good evidence that clogging of the arteries is reversible—if we take serious steps to control the disease process.'

Furthermore, I say: 'There's also good evidence to suggest that taking these steps will not only unclog the arteries but also lower one's risk of future heart attack and stroke. It's a win–win situation.'

Cardiovascular disease is preventable and can be controlled. This book is all about what can be done, how it can be done, and the tools we have to achieve these targets.

Unclog Your Arteries draws on my experience treating many hundreds of patients, who I believe have lived longer, healthier, more active and more rewarding lives because they have been able to control clogging of the arteries.

Part I discusses the arteries and how they become clogged, and what your risk factors are for the associated effects such as heart disease and stroke. Part II explains the facts of blood fats and demystifies cholesterol.

Part III covers lifestyle, and how what you eat, drink and do is reflected in your arteries, and how you can modify your behaviour to achieve artery health. In Part IV we start getting serious about what to do if you are diagnosed with clogged arteries and I take you through a program I have devised to help countless patients lower their risks of heart attack and stroke.

Of course, we all expect a magic bullet these days for instant health, and Part V gives you up-to-date information on modern medications and surgeries to clear and repair clogged arteries. In Part VI I discuss the treatment of clogged arteries for specific groups.

Making changes to the way you eat and cook is extremely important. Part VII includes valuable lessons on cooking with low-cholesterol, low-saturated fat ingredients.

In naming this book, I've decided to defer to my patients; it's what everyone wants to know: *how to unclog your arteries* and to keep those precious channels as clear as possible for the rest of your life.

Unclog Your Arteries has been written to help you understand how best to undertake a program to maintain optimal health and wellbeing. Your doctor will play an important role in this, because medications are an integral part of the anti-clogging program. As I said in my book *Men's Health*, however, knowledge is the key to an effective prevention program. Self-motivation is the other. The care and love of your spouse, partner, family or friends can also be a big factor in starting and maintaining this program. Good health!

Ian Hamilton-Craig

List of Acronyms and Common Terms

ACE inhibitor: Drug used to treat heart failure and blood pressure.

Adipose tissue: The fat layer under the skin and around the internal organs, comprising large cells filled with triglycerides (adipocytes).

Adventitia: The outermost layer of the wall of blood vessels.

Angina: Discomfort or pain in the chest, caused by lack of adequate blood supply to the heart muscle.

Angiogram: A diagnostic test in which dye is injected into an artery and X-rays are taken to determine the calibre of blood vessels.

Angioplasty: A procedure in which an inflatable balloon is threaded across an obstruction in a blood vessel, and the obstruction relieved by blowing up the balloon (see Stent).

Artery: A thick-walled blood vessel carrying blood away from the heart under relatively high pressure.

Arterioles: Small muscular arteries controlling the blood pressure level by their degree of contraction, and thereby peripheral resistance to blood flow.

Atherosclerosis: A chronic inflammatory disease involving all layers of the arterial wall, in which there is progressive thickening and cholesterol accumulation within the intima and narrowing of the lumen.

Blood pressure: The pressure exerted by the blood on the inner walls of the arteries, being relative to the force of the heartbeat and the elasticity and diameter of the blood vessels.

Body mass index (BMI): Body weight in kilograms divided by the square of the height in metres.

Capillaries: Very thin-walled blood vessels seen only with the microscope that allow diffusion of nutrients to the tissues from the blood and waste products from the tissues into the blood.

Cardiovascular diseases: Diseases of the heart and the blood vessels.

Coronary calcium score (CCS): Coronary clogging is related to the coronary calcium score (see page 35)

Cerebrovascular diseases: Diseases of the brain due to abnormal blood vessels.

Cholesterol: A fatty substance that is only made by animals and is a normal component of cell membranes, is a precursor to steroid hormones and bile acids, and is transported in the blood in lipoproteins.

Clot: A solid mass derived from coagulation of the blood outside the body.

Diabetes: A disease characterised by high blood glucose levels and premature clogging of the arteries.

Endothelial cells: Pavement-like cells lining the inner walls of arteries, veins and capillaries.

HDL (high density lipoproteins): Particles that transport cholesterol in the blood from the tissues to the liver, characterised by the presence of the protein apoA-1.

Hypertension: High blood pressure.

Infarct: An area of tissue that has died from lack of blood supply.

Intima: The inner layer of blood vessels.

LDL (low density lipoproteins): Particles that transport cholesterol in the blood from the liver to the tissues, characterised by the presence of the protein apoB-100 and derived from the metabolism of very low density lipoproteins.

Lipoproteins: Particles that transport fat in the blood.

Lumen: The central cavity within blood vessels that carries blood.

Macrophage: A cell involved in inflammation, derived from blood-borne monocyte, that may engulf cell debris and/or infectious particles.

Metabolic syndrome: A cluster of conditions that often occur together, including obesity, high blood sugar, high blood pressure and high triglycerides, which can lead to cardiovascular disease (also known as syndrome X or insulin resistance syndrome).

Monocyte: A white blood cell derived from the bone marrow, a precursor to tissue macrophages.

MRI (magnetic resonance imaging): Use of magnetic fields to visualize tissue structures through detection of variation in water content, which does not involve X-rays.

Myocardial infarction: Medical term for heart attack (see Infarct).

Patency: Degree to which the lumen of a blood vessel remains open (see Lumen).

Peripheral vascular disease: Atherosclerosis of the arteries to the limbs, head and neck.

Plaque: Area of accumulation of cholesterol and other substances in the inner lining of the arterial wall that may increase in size and obstruct blood flow.

Platelets: Blood cells that attach to sites of damage to blood vessels and are involved in thrombosis and coagulation (the solidification of blood).

Statin: Drug to lower LDL that partially inhibits the activity of a protein involved in the synthesis of cholesterol.

Stroke: Sudden loss of brain or nerve function caused by bleeding or infarction

Thrombolysis: The dissolution of a thrombus.

Thrombosis: The formation of a thrombus.

Thrombus: A solid mass, derived from coagulation of the blood in living blood vessels, formed from platelets, fibrin and other blood elements; may block a blood vessel at the place it formed.

Triglycerides: The storage form of fat, found in adipose tissue and transported in the blood within lipoproteins.

Part I

Of Arteries and Coronaries

This part explores exactly what we mean when we say clogged arteries or 'hardening of the arteries', and what the consequences are, such as heart attack and stroke.

1
What is Clogging of the Arteries?

The arteries of young children are 'as clean as a whistle'—like a newly laid garden pipe, their walls are smooth and shiny. With normal ageing, the walls do become a little thicker, but the blood channel remains just as open as it always was, so there is no impairment of blood flow to the tissues. This normal ageing process is called 'arteriosclerosis'.

In most Western societies, however, ageing of the body is accompanied by accumulation of cholesterol and other substances in the inner lining of the arteries, which become thickened to the extent that blood flow eventually becomes impaired, leading to heart attack, stroke, and several other diseases of the vascular system. This abnormal process is called 'atherosclerosis'—we'll simply call it clogging. It's analogous to the gradual rusting of iron pipes that carry water. As rusting proceeds, the flow of water is gradually impaired and can cut out altogether (see Figures 1.1 and 1.2).

Collaterals

Slow, gradual clogging of a single artery often has no symptoms and is a silent process; partly because the body can compensate through forming *collateral* channels, which function as natural bypasses.

Figure 1.1. Clogging of the arteries involves progressive, gradual thickening of the intima and impairment of blood flow.

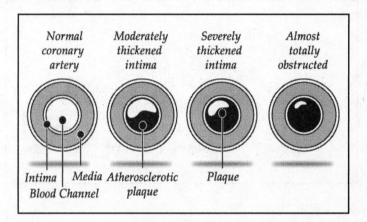

Figure 1.2. The silent—and deadly—progression of coronary clogging.

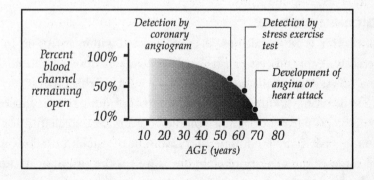

Collaterals are new vessels that allow blood to flow from a normal artery to another artery beyond a site of narrowing or obstruction

Plaque formation

The medical term for the abnormal tissue that accumulates in the wall of arteries as they become clogged is *atherosclerotic plaque*; we'll simply use the term 'plaque'. Figure 1.3 shows the structure of a plaque.

Figure 1.3. Structure of a plaque.

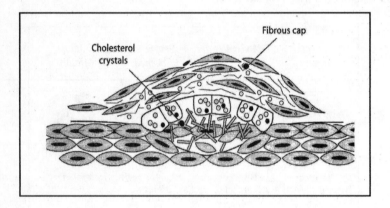

Plaques usually get bigger, often in an eccentric manner so that one side of the wall may be relatively normal while on the other side, the wall may become very thick.

Calcified plaques

Calcification is when calcium salts are deposited within any tissue. In the arterial wall, this process can be compared to what normally occurs in bone. Crystals of *calcium apatite* are formed during this process.

Calcification is an important component of plaques, and may account for up to 30 per cent of their volume. We can detect calcification by using special X-ray techniques. The amount of calcium used gives an indication of the severity of clogging as well as the risk of heart attack (see coronary calcium score, Chapter 3).

Clogging at different sites

Clogging may affect some arteries more severely than others for reasons we don't quite understand yet. Some factors seem to be more important for clogging at specific sites, as shown in Table 1.1.

Table 1.1 Factors associated with clogging of the arteries at different sites.

Risk factor	Coronary arteries	Brain arteries	Leg arteries
Cholesterol	+++	–	+
Blood pressure	+	+++	–
Smoking	++	–	+++

– minor association +++ major association

Coronary disease

The most common cause of heart attacks and sudden death is clogging of the coronary arteries. We'll discuss this further in Chapter 5: Heart Attack.

Cerebrovascular disease: Stroke

Stroke is one of the most-feared of illnesses because of the disabilities that may result—not only in performing skills but also in intellectual capacity and the resulting dependency on others.

There are several kinds of stroke, *cerebral infarction* being the most common. An infarct is an area of tissue that dies because of lack of blood supply; it can occur in almost any organ. Cerebral infarcts result when one of the arteries supplying blood to the brain is clogged.

Symptoms of stroke depend on which artery is involved. For example, middle cerebral artery occlusion may cause lack of movement and sensation on the other side of the body, with repercussions for speech and sight. These disabilities often improve in the weeks and months after the event.

High blood pressure and ageing are major risk factors for stroke, making it a common illness in the elderly.

Cholesterol is less powerfully related to cerebral infarction rates than blood pressure, but in spite of this, several trials of cholesterol-lowering with statins (drugs that lower cholesterol) have shown to reduce the risk of stroke and heart attack. The reason for this is not clear but may involve plaque stabilisation.

Cerebral haemorrhage is bleeding into the brain from a ruptured artery. It doesn't occur as often as cerebral infarction and is usually more severe—and more often fatal. Cerebral haemorrhage may cause extensive damage and brain swelling, with considerable disability. It is caused by high blood pressure, bleeding disorders, and rupture of cerebral aneurysms (sites of weakness in the artery wall which become ballooned out and are prone to rupture). High cholesterol levels are not related to cerebral haemorrhage.

Mini-strokes

The medical term for a mini-stroke is *transient ischaemic attacks* (TIAs). They are usually caused by clogging of the carotid arteries in the neck. There is a temporary loss of blood supply to an area of the brain or to the retina at the back of the eye. The sufferer will experience transient visual loss, weakness, or changes in sensation.

TIAs may be caused by bits of either cholesterol-rich plaque or blood clot on the surface of a plaque breaking off and travelling to the brain. These bits of tissue are called *emboli*. Anti-clotting treatment with aspirin may prevent TIAs due to clot emboli, and lowering cholesterol may stabilise plaques and reduce the tendency for cholesterol emboli to form.

Carotid plaques causing TIAs, or those of sufficient severity without symptoms, may also be treated surgically (*carotid endarterectomy*).

Clogging of the aorta and its branches in the abdomen

The aorta is the largest artery in the body. It arises from the heart and passes down alongside the spinal column in the chest into the abdomen, where it becomes the abdominal aorta. In the pelvis it divides into the iliac arteries, which supply blood to the pelvic organs and the buttock muscles. The iliac arteries then pass into the legs and become the femoral arteries (see Figure 1.4).

Figure 1.4 Clogging affects large arteries throughout the body.

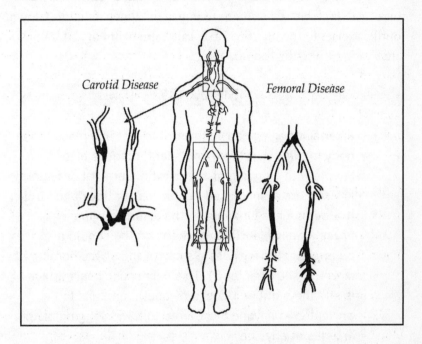

Clogging of these arteries may cause symptoms depending on where they are. Iliac disease may cause buttock pain on walking and erectile dysfunction. The abdominal aorta may become dilated because of ballooning out at an area of severe atherosclerosis and weakening of the vessel wall. The ballooned area is called an *aortic aneurysm*, and is prone to rupture.

Clogging of the arteries to the legs

Disease of the arteries to the legs (the femoral arteries) may cause *intermittent claudication:* pain in the calves on walking a certain distance, which is relieved rapidly by rest but recurs after walking the same distance. More severe narrowing may cause cold feet, ulceration of the toes and soles, and in its most severe stage, gangrene (death of tissues from lack of blood supply).

Disease in arteries to the kidneys and intestines

Occasionally, clogging of the arteries to the kidneys (*renal artery stenosis*) may cause high blood pressure and impaired kidney function. Clogging of the arteries to the intestines may cause intermittent abdominal pain after eating ('intestinal angina').

SUMMARY

- Arterial clogging causing symptoms at one place in the body implies that there are 'silent' plaques elsewhere.
- People with clogging of the carotid, cerebral or femoral arteries are at increased risk of heart attack and stroke.
- If a person has clogging of the arteries in the legs, brain, kidneys, aorta or neck, he or she should also be investigated for possible narrowing of the coronary arteries (see Chapter 5). This is because heart attack is still the number 1 cause of death, and has to be prevented in anyone discovered to have clogging of the arteries at any site.
- It is critical to control the risk factors for clogging, especially monitoring the blood fats *cholesterol* and *triglycerides* (see Chapter 8).
- Most people with clogging of the arteries also require a low dose of aspirin (75–100 mg daily is usual).

2
Plaques in the Arteries

Over many years of practice I have often seen arteries become un-clogged by examining repeat imaging studies of the arteries. It is a great sense of achievement for the patient and the doctor to literally be able to see this result in a test. Plaques really can shrink or actually disappear.

Figure 2.1 (over the page) shows a real case of unclogging plaques in the carotid artery (from 12-monthly ultrasound scans of the artery). The degree of clogging was reduced from 90 per cent to less than 80 per cent over a 12-month period of treatment with a cholesterol lowering drug, aspirin and medication to lower blood pressure.

Unclogging and drugs to lower cholesterol

Most studies of unclogging have involved treatment with powerful cholesterol-lowering drugs called *statins*, which mainly act to lower levels of the cholesterol fraction called LDL (see Chapter 8). Several different statins have been studied: lovastatin, pravastatin, simvastatin, fluvastatin, atorvastatin and rosuvastatin (see Chapter 28 for further details).

Less powerful LDL-lowering drugs have also been shown to unclog the arteries; some in combination with statins, including clofibrate, nicotinic acid, cholestyramine and colestipol (see Chapter 27).

The key element in unclogging the arteries is to lower LDL levels as far as possible (see Parts III and IV). Raising the good cholesterol fraction called HDL can also help.

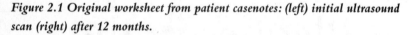

Figure 2.1 Original worksheet from patient casenotes: (left) initial ultrasound scan (right) after 12 months.

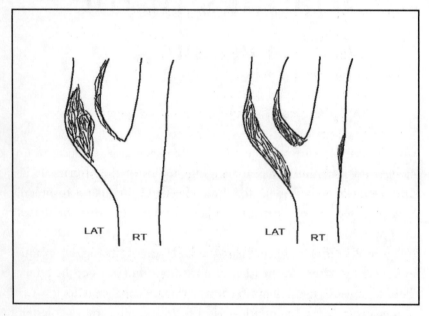

Clinical trials with the LDL-lowering drugs called statins (see Chapter 28) showed that statin treatment generally halted growth of existing plaques, prevented the formation of new plaques, and in some cases caused unclogging. The changes in plaque size were very small and were not expected to have much effect on either blood flow or numbers of heart attacks. It was therefore surprising that the numbers of heart attacks with statin treatment were reduced by up to 30 per cent compared with placebo.

The results of unclogging studies with statins have made us re-think the relationship of plaque severity (degree of narrowing) and the risk of having a heart attack. Most heart attacks occur because of rupture of relatively small plaques (less than 50 per cent narrowing of the artery). Our focus has now turned to trying to stabilise plaques and prevent them from rupturing. As a result, the risk of heart attacks and strokes will be considerably lower..

Other ways to help unclog the arteries

Other ways to help are to control key risk factors. They include:
- Quitting smoking (see Chapter 22)
- Eating LDL-friendly foods (see Part VII)
- Controlling blood pressure
- Getting as close to your ideal body weight as possible (see Chapter 20)

Fortunately, all these aims can be achieved by a single, simple approach: *Drive down the level of LDL and control key risk factors.* This book will show you how to do just that.

SUMMARY

- Controlling cholesterol (especially the LDL fraction) is important to unclog the arteries
- Other measures can also help: these include stopping smoking, a cholesterol-friendly diet, weight control and controlling blood pressure.
- Unclogging the arteries will reduce the risk of heart attack and stroke

3
What Causes Clogging?

Clogging of the arteries was first described in detail in the mid-19th century in Europe by German and Austrian pathologists, who first coined the term *atherosclerosis* to describe hardening of the arteries. They recognised that *sclerosis* (hardening) was accompanied by *athero*—from the Greek word meaning 'porridge'. This refers to the accumulation of a porridge-like soft material, which could be squeezed out from the vessel wall by firm pressure. The soft material was shown to contain large amounts of needle-like crystals of cholesterol, also visible under the microscope at the centre of plaques. They also observed other abnormalities, including areas of calcium deposition and fragmentation of the connective tissue fibres.

When fat stains were used to examine plaques, these scientists noticed large amounts of fat in the form of droplets at the sites of the porridge-like material. These droplets also occurred commonly within the muscle cells of the vessel wall and in large fat-filled cells with a foamy appearance—these cells were called *foam cells*. The chemical composition of fat droplets within the arterial wall was eventually defined. Without exception, they contained large quantities of cholesterol. Other substances were present in smaller amounts, including *phospholipids* (a fat that contains phosphorous) and *triglycerides*.

The severity of clogging, judged either by the degree of narrowing of the artery or by the area covered by plaques, was found to be proportional to the content of cholesterol in the vessel wall, as well as the blood cholesterol level. The obvious (and correct) interpretation of these facts is that cholesterol within the arterial wall is derived from cholesterol in the blood.

LDL and clogging

In the mid-1800s, the German pathologist Rudolf Virchow suggested that cholesterol in the blood filters into the arterial wall and causes clogging. It was a very astute observation for the time.

This concept is still valid, although not quite as simple. The blood component that delivers cholesterol to the arteries is called LDL (low density lipoprotein), also known as 'bad cholesterol' (see Chapter 8).

Under normal circumstances, cholesterol delivery is balanced by cholesterol removal through the action of HDL (high density lipoprotein), also called 'good cholesterol'.

Clogging of the arteries therefore occurs when there is an imbalance between LDL and HDL, causing cholesterol to accumulate in the arterial wall. Several factors may contribute to LDL/HDL imbalance, including:

- High blood levels of LDL
- Low blood levels of HDL
- High blood pressure
- Cigarette smoking
- Diabetes

Inflammation and clogging

Some years ago, I attended a medical conference in Canberra which looked at the pathology of clogging of the arteries. The purpose of the conference was to explore the possibility that clogging might be an inflammatory disease—a relatively new concept at the time.

The pathology of the atherosclerotic plaque was described in detail: *inflammatory cells* were always a prominent component of plaques. These cells were typical of those seen in a response to any immunological injury. It was suggested that perhaps infection or some other pro-inflammatory activator could result in vascular injury and therefore clogging.

Then, it was a rather off-beat concept but now there is considerable evidence that a low-grade ongoing inflammatory process occurs as clogging progresses. This is shown by increases in the blood levels of a variety of inflammatory markers, such as CRP (*C-reactive protein*).

Large population studies have shown that people with high levels of CRP also have higher rates of heart attack and are also the group with the best response to therapy with cholesterol-lowering drugs called statins (see Chapter 31).

The inflammatory markers may constitute a novel group of risk factors in the years ahead, which may be useful to discriminate people at higher risk of heart attack from those at lower risk.

CASE STUDY: TIM

Tim is a very good friend of mine. We went through university together, and have kept in touch ever since. Tim has been a busy GP for over 20 years, has kept reasonably fit, is a non-smoker, drinks lightly, and has virtually never had a day off in his life. Once a week he goes for a long walk with a lawyer friend and has a chance to talk about life, the universe, and anything of a non-medical nature.

After one walk he noticed he was more short of breath than usual, especially after climbing up an incline. His friend had no problem with the walk and Tim decided to put it out of his mind.

Next week the same thing happened, but Tim's symptoms were noticeably worse. He had no cough, or any other reason to think of a lung complaint. So he referred himself for an exercise stress test.

Halfway through the treadmill stages he again became noticeably short of breath but the ECG showed changes that indicated lack of blood supply to the heart muscle—the test was positive.

Tim's next test was a coronary angiogram. This showed significant narrowing of two out of three coronary arteries. The sites of narrowing were not suitable for balloon angioplasty and one week later Tim had a triple bypass operation.

Being a medico, he wanted to get to the science of the problem: 'Ian, I can't understand why this happened to me,' he said to me later. 'I have no risk factors. My cholesterol is normal, my HDL is normal, my triglycerides are normal, my LDL is normal. I'm a non-smoker, I'm not much overweight and I have no family history. Maybe I had some kind of an infection and if I had some courses of antibiotics, I wouldn't have developed coronary disease,' said Tim with his tongue only slightly in his cheek.

Tim's case is in fact quite uncommon. Recent studies have shown over 90 per cent of heart attack risk can be explained by nine easily measurable factors. In order of prediction, these are: high levels of cholesterol, cigarette smoking, diabetes, high blood pressure, abdominal obesity, psychological stress, low fruit and vegetable consumption, low physical exercise and low alcohol intake. These risk factors are discussed later in the book.

Five years on, I'm happy to report Tim is in good health and good spirits. He has modified his lifestyle (part-time work, less stress, more exercise and change in diet). With medication and careful medical supervision, he has every chance of seeing his grandchildren and watching them grow to adults.

Clotting and clogging

A *thrombus* is a solid tissue originating from components of the blood, formed within the living circulation. The process of thrombus formation is called *thrombosis*.

A blood clot, on the other hand, is a solid tissue formed in the test tube by *clotting*—coagulation of blood outside the living circulation.

Many doctors use the two terms interchangeably, although this is not strictly correct.

Thrombosis involves activation of tiny cells in the bloodstream called *platelets*, which stick together and release substances that transform a soluble protein into tiny interwoven strands, which surround clumps of platelets and red bloods cells, building into a solid mass—the thrombus.

Another mid-1800s German pathologist, Von Rokitansky, observed the occurrence of thrombi on the surface of plaques, and proposed that plaques could originate from thrombi.

Flowing blood creates strain at certain sites in the vascular system. Turbulent or irregular blood flow occurs particularly at vessel branches. A sequence of events may then follow in which platelets, the blood cells responsible for plugging leaks in the vascular system, release factors that can cause damage to the lining of the arteries and lead to clogging.

SUMMARY

- Clogging of the arteries involves many factors that can damage the lining and lead to cholesterol accumulation.
- LDL is a crucial component of the process.
- Thrombosis (blood clotting) may be involved in both the early and late stages of clogging the arteries.
- These complex mechanisms are amenable to drugs that block or modify the biochemical pathways involved, and can lower the risk of heart attack and stroke.

4
Getting Your Arteries Checked Out

One of the great dangers of clogging of the arteries is that there are often virtually no symptoms. It is a silent killer creeping along without any visible signs. So the clinician has to play detective and find out if clogging of the arteries is lurking around, how much there is and where—and then decide what to do about it.

The trouble is that up to the late stages of the disease, clogging in our arteries often builds up silently. Only those at the tip of the iceberg are aware of it through symptoms such as angina, or having suffered from heart attack. In an ideal world, we'd be able to identify all these with silent coronary disease, and treat them to prevent heart attack or the onset of symptoms. More importantly, we could prevent sudden death, which occurs in about one-third of those presenting for the first time with coronary symptoms.

Doctors and scientists have spent much time and effort looking at new ways to assess silent clogging. These days there are techniques that show promise, although research is in its early days and all these techniques are yet to be used in routine practice:

- CIMT (carotid artery intima-medial thickness)
- ABI (ankle-brachial blood pressure index)
- MRI (magnetic resonance imaging)
- CCS (coronary calcium score)

Carotid artery intima-medial thickness

The carotid arteries are very accessible as they lie just beneath the skin of the neck, just behind the angle of the jaw. They are easily examined with an ultrasound probe which can measure blood flow and the diameter of the carotid arteries.

The important measurement—as far as risk of cardiovascular disease is concerned—is the thickness of the intimal and medial layers (carotid intima-medial thickness, or CIMT). The CIMT slowly increases with ageing, but normally remains below 1.0 mm.

Clogging of the arteries is a generalised disease, and most large arteries throughout the body are usually affected to a similar degree. Changes in the carotid arteries can therefore indicate the condition of coronary and other arteries.

The American Heart Association has recommended CIMT measurement as an additional tool to assess coronary risk in people aged over 45 who are already at medium risk due to traditional risk factors. If someone showed a high CIMT, this would indicate the need for more aggressive treatment of risk factors—aiming for lower LDL and blood pressure levels.

CIMT is also a useful guide to the effectiveness of treatment. After effective cholesterol lowering, regression of both CIMT and carotid plaques can be shown by repeated carotid ultrasound studies (see case report and Figure 2.1).

CASE STUDY: JOHN

John, a 55-year-old car salesman, was found to have a CIMT of 0.9 mm (normal less than 0.7 mm) and an LDL of 4.5 (ideal 2.5 or less). After three years of treatment with a statin (drugs that lower LDL), in additional to a strict diet to lower LDL, his LDL fell to 1.8. Repeat carotid ultrasound showed improvement in CIMT to 0.6 mm, which is within the normal range.

There is no better evidence for the need to take tablets than seeing your own plaques get smaller or even disappear!

Ankle-brachial blood pressure index

Another relatively simple technique is measurement of systolic blood pressure in the upper arm and at the ankle. Systolic pressure is the higher of the two readings when blood pressure is taken. Normally, the systolic pressure at the upper arm is almost identical to that at the ankle, so the ratio of ankle/brachial pressure is 1.0. A low ratio is most commonly caused by obstruction to flow in the femoral artery in the thigh, where clogging is often quite severe.

An abnormal ABI is a signal that clogging is present at other sites: a low ABI (below 0.9) is associated with up to six times higher risk of heart attack and death, regardless of traditional risk factors.

Magnetic resonance imaging

Magnetic resonance imaging (MRI) has been available for several years and has been an extremely useful technique for imaging diseases of virtually every organ in the body.

MRI involves imaging the body's tissues through the use of a powerful magnetic field, and has the great advantage of being able to be repeated as often as necessary. In basic terms, the technique depends on the water content of the tissues and does not involve X-rays or any other potentially harmful radiation.

MRI has only recently been used to directly visualise the coronary arteries. This is because movement of the heart makes imaging very difficult unless images can be captured within fractions of a second.

It is only in recent years that rapid-speed MRIs have been constructed. RI appears to be the most promising tool for the future detection of silent clogging of the coronary arteries. It is currently available at relatively few centres.

Coronary calcium score

The principle behind the coronary calcium score (CCS) is that calcium is deposited during plaque evolution, as we have discussed in Chapter 1. Eventually, up to 30 per cent of plaque volume is made up of calcium salts. Calcium can be readily detected by X-rays because like bone it is very dense and does not let X-rays pass through.

A recent X-ray technique called computed tomography (CT) allows us to rapidly rotate an X-ray tube around the body, and generate cross-sectional images of any area that is a few millimetres in thickness. CT scans can examine cross-sections of the heart from top to bottom and any calcium within the coronary arteries can be detected. The amount of calcium in each section is added up to produce a coronary calcium score. The study of large numbers of people having both CCS and coronary angiography has related CCS to the severity of coronary clogging (see Table 4.1).

Table 4.1. Coronary clogging is related to the coronary calcium score

Coronary calcium score	Coronary plaque
0	None detected
1-10	Minimal plaque
11-100	Mild plaque
11-400	Moderate plaque
>400	Severe plaque with 50 per cent or more narrowing likely

Results can also be expressed in terms of *percentiles*. An average score is at the 50th percentile, a low score <25th percentile, and a high score >75th percentile. The CCS depends on age and gender. Men have significantly higher CCS than women, and CCS is higher with increasing age. Several studies have shown a relationship between CCS and risk of heart attack—the higher the CCS, the higher the risk.

It's been difficult to determine whether CCS responds to statin therapy. Some studies have shown increased CCS, while others have reduced CCS after several months of treatment, during which LDL levels were significantly lowered. With no treatment, CCS (when measured to indicate plaque volume) increases by up to 20–50 per cent annually.

There are several advantages to using CCS to detect silent coronary atherosclerosis:

- The technique uses routine CT equipment and is widely available.
- The cost has fallen considerably over the last few years and currently is about $AU200.
- No preparation is necessary (such as fasting).
- The test can take as little as 15 minutes to perform.

Many people come in for a heart scan with no previous symptoms, moderate levels of traditional risk factors, and have significantly high CCS (greater than 400 or the 75th percentile). These people need further investigation with exercise testing (treadmill test) and in some cases coronary angiography. Some require balloon angioplasty or bypass surgery to urgently unclog their arteries (see Chapter 33).

We still aren't sure for whom CCS is most appropriate as a screening test for silent coronary atherosclerosis. Authorities in the US have suggested that people with intermediate risk of heart attack based on traditional risk factors should be considered for the test.

Intravenous CT coronary angiography (CTCA)

Coronary angiography is an invasive technique in which a catheter is inserted into a femoral artery, threaded up to the coronary arteries via the aorta, and a contrast solution (opaque to X-rays) is then injected into each of the coronary arteries. Intravenous CT coronary angiography (CTCA) also uses contrast solution but this is injected into a vein in the forearm. X-rays and CT imaging are used to visualise the coronary arteries.

CTCA is very useful in people who have had previous coronary bypass surgery to see if the grafts are still open. These grafts are readily visualised with CTCA, and any blockages detected accurately. If narrowing or blockage has occurred, some grafts can be opened up by balloon angioplasty (see Chapter 33), while others may need repeat bypass surgery.

SUMMARY

- Silent clogging of the arteries is the enemy that needs to be conquered if we are to effectively prevent cardiovascular disease.
- The techniques described in this chapter are useful tests to help detect those at risk of cardiovascular disease.
- Their use is still under evaluation and with rapid improvements in technology, MRI scanning may become the method of choice in the not-too-distant future, but only at large centres because of the cost of installation.

5

Heart Attack

The two short words 'heart attack' frighten most people. The first thing we need to remember is that heart attack is not synonymous with death. Yes, some heart attacks are—tragically—fatal. But I have seen many patients who have lived through heart attack, learnt from the experience, and dealt so successfully with the health issues involved that they actually end up feeling better, stronger and more determined to combat the causes of the original attack.

People can and do recover from heart attack, as we'll discuss in this chapter. We'll also discuss the consequences of clogging of the coronary arteries: heart attack, angina and sudden death. Let's start with an anatomy lesson on the coronary arteries.

Coronary arteries

The two coronary arteries (left and right) supply blood to the heart muscle, and originate from the aorta. Then they travel downward over the surface of the heart and branch into smaller vessels. Eventually their branches penetrate into the heart muscle and very small vessels come into contact with muscle cells (see Figure 5.1).

Obstruction to blood flow

Unfortunately, clogging of the arteries is what I call a silent killer. Some people die suddenly from clogging of the coronary arteries without ever having experienced a single episode of chest pain or other classic symptoms of heart disease.

Others are in some ways more fortunate, because they develop symptoms leading to admission to hospital and treatment. I sometimes tell these patients they are the lucky ones, because they have been given a warning and can make lifestyle changes, take medication and be controlled in order to prevent further problems.

Figure 5.1. The normal coronary arteries.

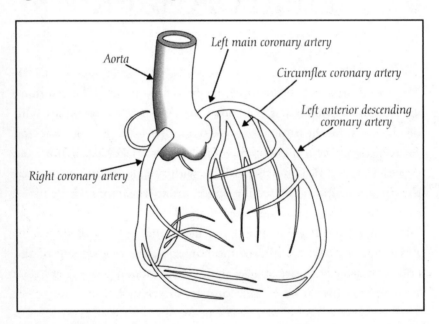

Coronary clogging can cause problems in two ways:

1. Gradual obstruction of blood flow

In this case, the area allowing blood to flow past becomes progressively smaller, rather like the silting up of a rusty pipe. At a critical point of obstruction (when the diameter of the passage has been narrowed by more than 75 per cent), any further reduction in blood flow leads to lack of oxygen supply to the heart muscle. A gradual reduction in flow causes a *collateral circulation* ('nature's bypass') to form. This is when new blood vessels grow from one side of the blockage to the other, allowing blood to flow around the obstruction. Think of it as like new channels forming in a river to bypass an obstacle.

This is our body's way of compensating for a severely obstructed vessel through developing alternative channels. For this reason, slowly progressive narrowing of the coronary arteries often occurs silently, without symptoms, and may not result in any heart damage.

2. Sudden obstruction of blood flow

In this case, an atherosclerotic plaque suddenly ruptures and exposes circulating blood to the highly thrombogenic (clot-promoting) contents of the plaque. A thrombus or clot (solid mass of blood cells enmeshed by filaments of the protein *fibrin*) rapidly forms, suddenly reducing blood flow to the heart muscle.

Outcome and symptoms of gradual obstruction

There may be no symptoms if collateral channels are sufficiently well developed. In other cases, for example during unaccustomed exercise (such as pushing a stalled car), nerves from the heart are stimulated by lack of oxygen and one can experience dull, central chest ache or tightness. This symptom is called *angina* and is alleviated quickly by resting.

Heart failure is another complication of severe progressive narrowing of the coronary arteries. This happens when the pumping action of the heart is impaired as a result of inadequate blood supply. The symptoms include fatigue, weakness and shortness of breath, especially during exercise.

Outcome and symptoms of sudden obstruction

Sudden obstruction to flow is very dangerous because there are no collateral channels to compensate. The muscle can survive for only a few minutes without oxygen and the other nutrients it normally receives from arterial blood. Depending on the severity and site of the obstruction, the condition of the heart muscle, and other factors, very different outcomes may result. These include:

- Unstable angina
- Heart attack
- Sudden death

1. Unstable angina

With less than 100 per cent obstruction, there is enough blood to keep the heart muscle alive, and heart muscle becomes *hypoxic* (with less than adequate oxygen).

Pain fibres supplying the heart muscle are stimulated by hypoxia, causing anginal pain. This is often more severe than in the case of gradual obstruction. Sufferers describe the sensation as a 'crushing', 'burning' or 'vice-like' pain, or 'heaviness'. The sufferer will often feel the pain in their sternum, at the centre of the chest; they may mistake it for a bad case of indigestion.

The sufferer may experience the pain elsewhere, depending on which part of the heart muscle is affected and the segment of the spinal cord that sends out pain fibres to the area. Pain arising from one area can be experienced in another place if it has the same segmental innervation from the spinal cord (a phenomenon called *radiation* of pain). For example, if the diaphragm below the heart is irritated, the sufferer may experience this as shoulder-tip pain, because both areas have the same segmental nerve supply.

Angina can therefore be experienced as pain (or tightness, heaviness, burning or similar sensation) in either the chest, shoulder, neck, jaw, teeth, arms, elbow, wrist, fingers, abdomen or back. The diagnosis of angina may not therefore be straightforward. Other tests are often necessary.

One of the clues to a correct diagnosis of angina is if the pain is relieved by administering *glyceryl trinitrate* (GTN), either in the form of a spray under the tongue, a tablet kept under the tongue until it dissolves, or in an intravenous drip. GTN is a powerful dilator of blood vessels, and may improve blood supply to hypoxic heart muscle, thereby relieving anginal pain.

Angina due to sudden obstruction is called 'unstable' because it may change its character and severity quite quickly and there is a high risk that it will develop into a heart attack if further obstruction occurs.

For these reasons, people with recent-onset, new or a different kind of angina from what they usually experience are admitted to hospital and closely monitored and investigated. Coronary angiography is often performed to see where the obstruction is and what can be done to relieve it.

2. Heart attack

With 100 per cent obstruction, the affected area of heart muscle becomes dysfunctional. It can't contract properly. As a result, cells begin to die from complete lack of oxygen (*anoxia*). The area that has died from lack of blood supply is called an *infarct*. A heart muscle infarct is called a *myocardial infarction.*

Heart attacks are most common in older people, particularly between the ages of 50 and 75 (see Figure 5.2), which I call the 'danger years'. The rates in younger women are relatively low compared with men of the same age.

Overall, two men are admitted to hospital with heart attack for every woman admitted, although the death rate is similar in men and women, and rises dramatically with increasing age. The most likely explanation for this is the gradual progression of coronary atherosclerosis, as all major coronary vessels narrow as we get older. Sudden blockage of a major coronary artery is more likely to cause death if the other coronary arteries are severely narrowed, as is often the case in the elderly.

Heart attack causes severe central chest pain, often described as crushing or vice-like in nature. The symptoms are similar to those of unstable angina but are often more severe, prolonged, and unlike unstable angina, are not relieved by GTN. Like unstable angina, heart attack pain can be misdiagnosed as indigestion, or shoulder trouble, or back pain, or gall bladder disease, or one of several other disorders.

Figure 5.2. Age and gender of patients admitted to hospital with heart attack.

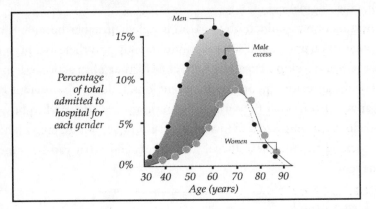

Heart attack pain is often associated with sweating, nausea and a feeling of impending death. The sufferer may experience light-headedness and giddiness, and may collapse in unconsciousness. About one person in ten does not survive the first few weeks following the onset of chest pain. Chest pain often requires further investigation to figure out the cause. Initially, we perform an ECG (electrocardiogram) and blood tests to measure levels of a protein called *troponin* that is released by damaged heart muscle.

3. Sudden death

In the worst-case scenario, sudden death may occur from an unexpected obstruction as a result of electrical instability that interrupts the normal automatic pacemaker activity of the heart. An abnormal heart rhythm called *ventricular fibrillation* occurs. This interrupts the muscle function of the heart and leads to cardiac arrest. With no blood supply to the body's tissues (especially the brain) from a heart that has ceased to beat, the sufferer can die within minutes. In up to one-third of cases, sudden death is the first sign of underlying coronary disease. Some people can be resuscitated, but most are unable to be revived because of the delay in starting treatment.

Recovery from acute obstruction

Following a heart attack, over a period of up to three weeks, scar tissue replaces areas of dead heart muscle. During this period of healing, areas of undamaged heart muscle take over the function of the heart and remodelling begins, in which there are changes in the size and shape of the heart. Most people make a good recovery after heart attack and many can return to normal life. Remodelling doesn't occur after unstable angina because a large area of heart muscle hasn't died, as is the case during heart attack.

Acute coronary syndrome

Unstable angina and heart attack may be difficult to distinguish in the early phases. A person admitted to hospital with chest pain is given the diagnostic label of *acute coronary syndrome* (ACS).

SUMMARY

- Heart attacks occur with sudden obstruction of flow within the coronary arteries, causing death of heart muscle.
- The underlying cause of obstruction is plaque rupture, followed by thrombosis (blood clotting) at the surface and within the plaque.
- Sudden death can occur from electrical instability of the heart, especially within the first hour after the onset of symptoms, and may be the first evidence of clogging of the arteries in up to one-third of cases.
- Gradual obstruction of coronary flow can allow the development of collateral channels ('nature's bypasses'), maintaining blood flow to the heart muscle and preventing symptoms. Silent, progressive clogging will eventually narrow the blood channel.

6
Risk Factors for Heart Attack and Stroke

Doctors often use the term *risk factor*. A risk factor is a predictor of future disease. For example, smokers are more likely to get lung cancer than non-smokers; therefore smoking is a risk factor for lung cancer. Smoking is also a risk factor for heart attack and stroke, and is one of the first things to eliminate in any healthy lifestyle program.

Risk factors for heart attack and stroke were first defined in the early 1950s by researchers at Framingham, a small town of about 5000 people near Boston. These researchers decided to carry out a survey of the entire adult population, and measured all the factors that were thought at the time to be related to heart attack or stroke. Since then, the townsfolk have been checked annually for almost 50 years. Those suffering from heart attack or stroke were studied further to analyse any possible relationship between the initial measurements and the subsequent development of disease. This has led to the description of risk factors, which predict the likelihood of occurrence of diseases, including coronary heart disease and stroke. Risk factors for heart attack and stroke can be classified as either non–modifiable (ones we can't change) or modifiable (ones we can change). The coronary risk factors we cannot change include:

- **Gender:** Heart attack is more common in men than women. This is especially so for premenopausal women, who have one-fifth the heart attack fatality rate of men. After the menopause, women almost catch up with men. In their early seventies, women have half the rate of men, and over age 85 rates are similar in men and women (see Figure 6.1).

- **Age:** Increasing age is one of the most powerful risk factors. Mortality rates are very low below the age of 50, and greatly increase with age, as shown in Figure 6.1.

- **Family history:** Risk is increased if other family members have suffered heart attack, especially in parents or siblings before the age of 55 in men and 65 in women.

Figure 6.1. Heart attack fatality rates according to age and gender.

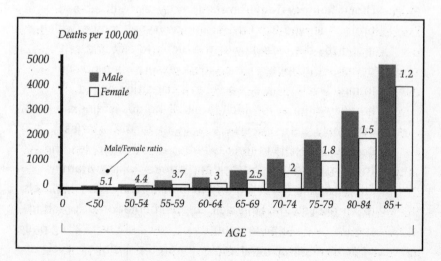

The coronary risk factors we can control and change include:

- **Blood fat levels:** As we have seen in previous chapters, heart attack risk is greater with increasing levels of cholesterol, LDL and triglycerides—high levels of these blood fats are harmful. The opposite applies for HDL, high levels of which are protective.

- **Blood Lp(a):** This is a particle in the blood that also carries a small amount of cholesterol, and is related structurally to LDL. Like LDL, it can deliver cholesterol to the arteries and if levels are high, can contribute to clogging of the arteries. High Lp (a) levels are inherited.

- **Cigarette smoking:** Smoking doubles risk compared with non-smokers.

- **Blood pressure:** Risk increases with increasing blood pressure. This relationship applies to both kinds of blood pressure that are routinely measured: the higher systolic pressure and the lower diastolic pressure.

- **Weight:** Increased risk occurs in those with central (abdominal) obesity when abdominal fat accumulates (see Chapter 20).

- **Physical exercise:** Sedentary habits increase coronary risk.

- **Blood homocysteine level:** Homocysteine is a blood protein derived from the amino acid methionine, which increases the tendency of the blood to clot and can damage the lining of the blood vessels when present in high levels. There is a genetic condition called homocystinuria, in which levels of homocysteine are extremely high, and severe clogging of the arteries occurs in people in their twenties and thirties, leading to premature heart attack and stroke. Taking vitamin supplements (B12, B6 and folic acid) can lower the levels of homocysteine. Folic acid supplementation of bread in the US by as small a quantity of folic acid as 0.2 mg daily appears to have significantly lowered population levels of homocysteine, and may have contributed to the lower rate of heart attacks seen over the last few years.

- **Blood C-reactive protein level:** Doctors in the US are now using measurement of C-reactive protein (CRP) to help estimate heart attack risk. CRP is an index of inflammation, and can be raised in many diseases, especially infections. High CRP levels have been shown to be linked with increased heart attack risk in several large US studies.
- **Diabetes mellitus:** Diabetes doubles the risk of heart attack in men and increases risk up to four-fold in women.
- **Impaired kidney function and after kidney transplantation:** Heart attack is more frequent in people with kidney disease, partly as a result of abnormal blood fats, but also other co-existing risk factors including high blood pressure.
- **Previous vascular disease:** Heart attack and stroke risk is increased with previous heart attack, bypass surgery, stroke, clogging of the carotid arteries in the neck and of the femoral arteries in the leg.
- **Thickening of the heart muscle:** This usually occurs as a result of long-standing high blood pressure, and doubles risk of heart attack. Thickening of the heart muscle alters the electrical signals from the heart and can be detected on an electrocardiogram (ECG). It can also be detected by ultrasound examination (echocardiogram).

Since the 1950s, over 100 risk factors have been described, including high blood levels of uric acid, abnormalities in the levels of various clotting factors, and the presence of albumin in the urine that may reflect kidney damage.

High blood pressure
The blood vessels, especially the arteries, are designed to withstand the

pressure of the blood flowing inside. For this reason they have thick layers of elastic and collagen fibres, which stretch and recoil with each heartbeat, protecting the vessel wall from undue stresses and strains.

High blood pressure alters this dynamic. The stresses and strains on the vessel wall are greatly accentuated, causing damage to the lining. This is particularly the case at branching points where flow becomes turbulent, allowing greater interaction between blood cells, and greater injury to the delicate cells that line the vessel walls.

If you look at a bend in a wide, slowly flowing river, you will see sand accumulating on the inside of the bend, and also on both sides of the river beyond the bend. This model illustrates what happens in our arteries as a result of the curves and branches. High blood pressure accentuates these changes.

Basically, if you have high blood pressure, you double your risk of stroke and heart attack. If you also have high cholesterol, your risk is increased even more (depending on how high your cholesterol is).

The good news is: by simply lowering blood pressure, you reduce your risk of heart attack and stroke. As is the case for cholesterol, there is no lower limit to this benefit. 'The lower the better' generally applies to blood pressure, with the proviso that if blood pressure is lowered too much, one can get giddy on sudden standing, and excessively low blood pressure can adversely affect kidney and heart function.

About 20 per cent of the adult population has high blood pressure. The percentage rises with increasing age so about 50 per cent of the elderly have high blood pressure.

The number of risk factors doubles your risk

Note this very important concept: risk factors are *multiplicative* rather than additive. This effectively means that where there is one additional risk factor, risk is doubled. Two additional risk factors increase risk almost four times. Three additional risk factors (such as smoking, high cholesterol and high blood pressure) increases risk almost nine times.

Association with heart disease—but not the cause

If a given risk factor is related to heart attack or stroke, it does not necessarily mean that the factor itself causes these diseases. It may only be a 'marker' (innocent bystander). A given risk factor is likely to cause a heart attack or stroke if there is a plausible biological mechanism evident that can also be tested and verified by scientific experiment. Causative risk factors include:

- High LDL, which leads to cholesterol accumulation in the arterial wall.
- Low HDL, which impairs removal of cholesterol from the arterial wall, and impairs other protective actions (see Chapter 9).
- High blood pressure, which damages the lining of the arteries.
- Cigarette smoking, which also damages the lining of the arteries.

SUMMARY

- Risk factors can be modifiable or non-modifiable.
- Risk factors are *multiplicative* rather than additive.
- Risk factors demonstrate *association* not *causation*.
- Risk factor control has been shown to reduce rates of cardiovascular disease.

In the next chapter, you will be able to measure your own risk for heart attack and stroke from a variety of sources, including the Framingham study.

7
Measuring Your Risk of Heart Attack and Stroke

Now that we have explored risk factors, we can learn how they can be used to predict the possibility of future disease, and to plan a campaign to control clogging of the arteries.

Like a good military general, the doctor has to understand the strength of the enemy forces in order to marshal his or her resources and to mount a counter-attack.

Today we do have the weapons to fight heart disease, so it is just a matter of planning the campaign, and putting it into action.

When we predict future diseases (otherwise known as risk assessment) we use a combination of several risk factors, such as age and blood pressure, in order to assess the likelihood of developing heart attack or stroke at some time in the future. Risk assessment uses a combination of all the traditional risk factors to obtain an overall assessment of risk. This is called estimation of *global risk*.

Global risk

The following risk factors are usually included in measuring risk:
- Age
- Gender
- Either LDL or total cholesterol level
- HDL level
- Triglycerides (fasting level)
- Diabetes
- Cigarette smoking
- Blood pressure (systolic and/or diastolic level)
- Family history of heart disease

According to recent surveys, these risk factors are very common, especially in older age groups:
- High cholesterol (5.5 or above) occurs in 51 per cent of men and women.
- High triglycerides (2.0 or above) occurs in 25 per cent of men and 17 per cent of women.
- Diabetes occurs in 8 per cent of men and 7 per cent of women.
- High blood pressure occurs in 31 per cent of men and 27 per cent of women.
- 18 per cent of men and 13 per cent of women are smokers.
- About 7 per cent of the population takes drugs to lower blood fats.

How to estimate risk of heart attack and stroke

Methods include:
- Entering data straight into the computer either using a personal 'risk-disc' or the internet
- Using graphs
- Using colour charts

How to estimate your 10-year risk of heart attack

Add up your points from the following tables:

1. AGE (YEARS)	Points	
	Men	Women
20–34	–9	–7
35–39	–4	–3
40–44	0	0
45–49	3	3
50–54	6	6
55–59	8	8
60–64	10	10
65–69	11	12
70–74	12	14
75–79	13	16

2. TOTAL CHOL	Points				
Cholesterol	20-39 yrs men wmn	40-49 men wmn	50-59 men wmn	60-69 men wmn	70-79 men wmn
less than 4.1	0 0	0 0	0 0	0 0	0 0
4.1–5.1	4 4	3 3	2 2	1 1	0 1
5.2–6.1	7 8	5 6	3 4	1 2	0 1
6.2–7.2	9 11	6 8	4 5	2 3	1 2
7.2 or more	11 13	8 10	5 7	3 4	1 2

Note: Use average of two previous measurements if possible.

3. HDL	Points—men and women
1.6 or above	–1
1.3–1.5	0
1.0–1.2	1
Less than 1.0	2

Note: Use average of two previous measurements if possible.

4. CIGARETTE SMOKING	Points								
Habit	20–39 yrs men wmn		40–49 men wmn		50–59 men wmn		60–69 men wmn		70–79 men wmn
Non-smoker	0	0	0	0	0	0	0	0	0	0
Smoker	8	9	5	7	3	4	1	2	1	1

Note: A smoker is anyone who has smoked in the last month.

5. SYSTOLIC BLOOD PRESSURE	Points			
SBP	Untreated men	wmn	Treated men	wmn
Less than 120	0	0	0	0
120–129	0	1	1	3
130–139	1	2	2	4
140–159	1	3	2	5
160 or above	2	4	3	6

What's your score?

10-year risk of heart attack is determined by the total point score. Very high risk is 20% or above; high risk is 15-19%, moderate is 10-14%, mild is 5-9% and low risk is less than 5%.

10-YEAR RISK %														
Points	0	1–4	5–6	7	8	9	10	11	12	13	14	15	16	17+
Men %	<1	1	2	3	4	5	6	8	10	12	16	20	25	30+
Women %	<1	1	2	3	4	5	6	8	11	14	17	22	27	30+

Note: This table only estimates risk. Your measurement will be more accurate if you include more risk factors in the equation, such as family history, diabetes and fasting triglycerides. See www.chd–taskforce.com for more detailed tables.

Websites for estimation of risk

Australia

National Heart Foundation/Cardiac Society of Australia and New Zealand: **www.heartfoundation.com.au**

Europe

Task Force on Coronary Prevention: **www.chd-taskforce.com**
Joint British Societies coronary risk prediction chart:
www.hyp.ac.uk/bhs/riskpv.htm
Risk prediction in adults with high blood pressure:
www.riskscore.org.uk
This website estimates five-year heart attack and stroke risk using the traditional risk factors as well as height and kidney function.

United States
American Heart Association: **www.americanheart.org**

This website estimates ten-year coronary risk from traditional risk factors as does the NCEP website below.
National Cholesterol Education Program:
www.nhlbi.nih.gov/guidelines/cholesterol/atp_iii.htm
This has a ten-year coronary risk calculator; use online or download.

New Zealand

New Zealand Cardiovascular Risk Calculator: **www.nzgg.org.nz**
The easy-to-use, colour-coded chart has certain advantages over other risk estimators:
- It includes HDL.
- It estimates risk for stroke as well as heart attack.
- It applies to a wide range of ages and risk factors.
- It includes diabetes.
- Global risk is based on the Framingham population, whose risk profile is similar to that of many other Western countries.

The NZ charts use total/HDL cholesterol ratio, which is a convenient way to describe the opposite effects of total cholesterol (equivalent to LDL) and HDL.

In Chapter 9, we learn that high levels of cholesterol and LDL are associated with higher risk and high levels of HDL are linked with lower risk. The Framingham study, in fact, was the first to show that total/HDL cholesterol ratio was a more powerful predictor of cardiovascular disease than either LDL or HDL alone. The benefits of treatment for people at various risk levels are shown in Table 7.1.

Table 7.1. Benefits of treatment for cardiovascular disease

Risk level (5-year risk of cardio-vascular disease)	Events prevented per 100 treated for 5 years*	Number needed to treat for 5 years to prevent 1 event*
Greater than 30 per cent	More than 10	Less than 10
25–30 per cent	9	11
20–25 per cent	7.5	13
15–20 per cent	6	16
10–15 per cent	4	25
5–10 per cent	2.5	40
2.5–5 per cent	1.25	80
Less than 2.5 per cent	Less than 0.8	More than 120

It is important to note that the NZ risk estimator can't be used for those who have already had a heart attack, stroke or other cardiovascular disease. These people are automatically placed in a high-risk category (more than 20 per cent risk of cardiovascular disease in five years). They also do not apply to those who have genetically high cholesterol, or those with extreme levels of any single risk factor (for example, those at the highest blood pressure levels). These people are at higher risk than the chart estimates. Other people whose risk may be underestimated by the New Zealand charts include:

- The presence of thickening of the heart muscle (usually from high blood pressure)—risk is greater than 20 per cent in five years.
- A strong family history of cardiovascular disease in first-degree relatives (parents, siblings or children). This applies to cardiovascular disease before age 55 in men and 65 in women.*
- Very high cholesterol (over 8.5).*
- Very high blood pressure (over 170/100).*
- Very obese (body mass index more than 30; this is height in (space) cm divided by the square of weight in (space) kg)*.

* In these cases, risk should be increased by at least one colour category on the NZ Cardiovascular Risk Calculator. Note that the point-scoring system derived from the Framingham study estimates *heart attack* risk rather than risk of *heart attack + stroke* given by the NZ charts.

SUMMARY

- We can estimate risk of heart attack and stroke using a variety of tools, but these assessments must be regarded as only an *approximation* of the real risk because the tables, charts and figures used are based on clinical trials of limited duration and in limited numbers of people.
- Nevertheless, measuring global risk remains an important method to determine outlook, and is a guide to how we can control blood fats and other risk factors (see Parts III-IV).
- The New Zealand charts are recommended as they include risk of stroke and heart attack.

Part II

All About
Blood Fats

In this part, I discuss cholesterol and other fats
found in the blood—and how they contribute
to clogged arteries and coronary disease.

8
Cholesterol, Triglycerides and Lipoproteins

Imagine tiny particles swirling around in the bloodstream, knocking into each other and exchanging bits of their surface material as cholesterol moves from one particle to another and back again.

Now think of those billions of muscle cells, or nerve cells, or heart cells, or liver cells. Each of these cells is surrounded by a membrane, like a cellophane wrapper, that is rich in cholesterol. The cholesterol plays an important role in maintaining normal function of the membrane, for example its ability to act as a barrier to certain substances, and not to others. A very important fact to remember is that cholesterol in the body is not an inert substance. It is part of the dynamism of life; a given molecule of cholesterol in a relatively fixed cell membrane is constantly being replaced by another, or taken into the interior of the cell, or gobbled up by particles in the bloodstream.

By contrast, cholesterol in the test tube is a white powder. Add water, and the cholesterol floats to the surface rather like talcum powder, showing that cholesterol is insoluble in water. Add, instead, a fat solvent such as acetone, and the white powder dissolves into a colourless solution.

Cholesterol in the body rarely exists as pure cholesterol because of its water insolubility. Instead, cholesterol is packaged with other molecules into several important body components:

- **Cell membranes** are like cellophane wrappers surrounding each of the body's cells. Each cell membrane is only a few millionths of a millimetre thick, and if you could enlarge it enough, it would look something like a sandwich. Cholesterol is a key component of cell membranes, and is therefore essential for living cells to function normally.
- **Lipoproteins** are tiny particles that transport cholesterol in the blood. These particles vary in size and have an outer skin and an inner core like miniature grapefruit, oranges, limes and lemons. Lipoproteins are classified according to their size and density, and we'll look at them in more detail in Chapter 9.
- **Cholesterol attached to transport proteins.** Cholesterol can be transported across cell membranes by attaching to proteins.

The worst thing about cholesterol is its stealth—we are unaware that it's there, building up in our arteries, increasing its lethal potential. Cholesterol can accumulate within the walls of the body's arteries and lead to clogging of the arteries, as discussed in Chapter 1. Clogging causes gradual blockage of the large arteries of the body, especially those supplying the heart muscle, brain, legs and kidneys.

Triglycerides: The forgotten fats

Most people these days are familiar with the word cholesterol and recognise that it is a major health issue; however, this wasn't the case when I first started to practise cardiology. These days we see 'low-cholesterol' products in the supermarket, we read about it in the press, we hear discussions about it on the radio, and we see stories about it on TV. Cholesterol is a buzz-word of our times and people discuss their cholesterol levels in the same way as they talk about their golf handicaps.

But very few people know about triglycerides. Yet these are very important; indeed, we cannot talk about clean, clear, healthy arteries without being aware of what triglycerides are and what they do.

The fat under the skin of animals and birds is largely made of triglycerides. This word is derived from the chemical structure of triglycerides: three fatty acid molecules are joined to a backbone of glycerol.

Fatty acids are long chains, 16–20 carbon atoms in length, which vary in shape and structure depending on the length of the chain and the number of double bonds, which allow the chains to bend.

Whalers in the 1800s were very aware of the importance of the layer of fat under the whale's skin—blubber—that insulated the whale against the cold, and also served as an energy source for the whale's metabolism. Blubber was melted down in enormous vats and whale oil transported back in barrels to Europe and America where its controlled combustion kept the lights burning and warmed many thousands of homes for almost 50 years, until fossil-based fuels became available.

Triglycerides as a source of energy
Like whale blubber, fat under the skin of animals, birds and fish can be burned slowly to provide energy for the various metabolic reactions of the body, as well as providing heat to maintain body temperature.

Triglyceride fatty acids
Let's return to the three fatty acids that make up each triglyceride molecule. Depending on the type and number of links between the carbon atoms, fatty acids can be either:
  * saturated

- monounsaturated
- polyunsaturated

Saturated fatty acids typically occur in fats of animal origin, including dairy foods (cheese, milk and butter) and visible fats in meat.

Monounsaturated fatty acids typically occur in certain plant fats (oils such as olive and canola and nuts such as macadamias).

Polyunsaturated fatty acids typically occur in plant oils (such as safflower and sunflower), as well as fish oils. Fish oils are also called *omega-3* fatty acids because of their unique structure.

By varying the proportions of these different types of fatty acids, triglycerides may differ in physical properties and appearance:

Saturated fats make triglycerides solid at room temperature (cheese and butter are good examples).

Polyunsaturated and monounsaturated fats make triglycerides liquid at room temperature (corn, safflower and olive oils).

Blood triglycerides

In the fasting state, blood triglycerides are much lower than cholesterol, and vary between 0.5 and 2.0.

Soon after a meal, however, triglyceride levels are much higher because dietary fats from the intestine are absorbed. High triglycerides persist for several hours, until they are cleared from the blood, when fasting levels are restored.

To prevent food interfering with the fasting levels of triglycerides, it is necessary to fast for at least 12 hours before taking blood to measure blood fat levels. You can do this with an overnight fast. During this time you can drink water (but don't have sugar as sugar can raise blood triglyceride levels).

Triglycerides, heart disease and stroke

Triglycerides play a key role in diseases such as obesity, diabetes and heart disease; we'll discuss this in later chapters.

SUMMARY

- Cholesterol is a naturally occurring fat that is not soluble in water unless physically associated with water-soluble substances such as phospholipids and proteins. It is essential to life.

- Excessive levels of cholesterol in the blood cause cholesterol to accumulate in the arteries, which can lead to heart attack and stroke.

- Triglycerides are essential body components that act as an energy storehouse, supplying fatty acids that can be burned by the body to supply energy for metabolism.

- Triglycerides play an important role in obesity, diabetes and heart disease, as we shall see later.

- The blood contains microscopic particles of fat called lipoproteins that transport fat to and from the liver. There are several types; all play a key role in delivering cholesterol to the arterial wall and removing it.

- An imbalance in blood cholesterol and/or triglycerides may have dire consequences—especially clogging of the arteries.

9
Good and Bad Cholesterol

Tracking cholesterol is like a medical detective story, and like all detective stories there are the Goodies and the Baddies. We have learnt that cholesterol is not a foreign substance in the body. It is a vital, necessary part of life. You can't live without it. But there is good and bad cholesterol and it is important to be able to distinguish between them.

The good cholesterol—HDL

In the 1950s, medical researchers at Framingham, near Boston, were the first to show that high cholesterol levels increase our risk of heart attack. At the same time, researchers in California were also studying risk factors for coronary heart disease, but had more sophisticated methods to measure cholesterol within the various lipoprotein fractions, including LDL and HDL. They drew a link between LDL cholesterol levels and risk of coronary heart disease (see Figure 9.1).

For this reason, LDL cholesterol is called 'bad' cholesterol. From now on we'll simply call it LDL.

Figure 9.1. Heart attack rates increase with increasing levels of LDL.

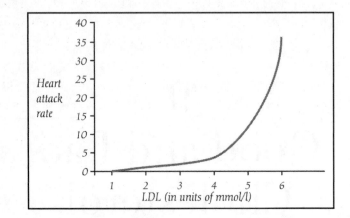

To their surprise, the Californian group also found that cholesterol in the HDL fraction had the opposite relationship to LDL. In other words, low levels of HDL cholesterol (which we'll call HDL) were associated with a high risk of heart attack, and high levels of HDL were linked with low risk (see Figure 9.2). HDL cholesterol is 'good' cholesterol.

Figure 9.2. Heart attack rates are lower with increasing levels of HDL.

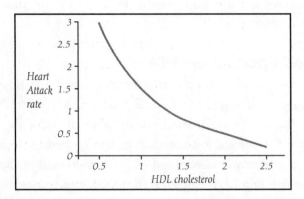

The significance of this discovery was not realised until the mid-1970s, when other researchers confirmed the relationship between higher HDL levels and a reduced risk of heart attack.

Why is HDL protective?

One reason for the protective effects of HDL is that HDL can pick up cholesterol from the arterial wall and return it to the liver for excretion from the body via the bile after conversion to bile acids.

The rate of cholesterol accumulation in arteries therefore depends on the balance between blood levels of LDL (bad cholesterol) and HDL (good cholesterol). As we've seen, these levels have opposite effects on our risk of coronary disease.

One convenient way to incorporate the opposite risks of HDL and LDL into a single number is to calculate the LDL/HDL ratio. This varies from about 1.0 at birth to over 30.0 in very rare cases of genetic high blood cholesterol levels. Populations with ratios below 2.5 have low rates of heart attack, while those with ratios of 5.0 or above have high rates of heart attack. Let's look at some high-risk and low-risk cholesterol profiles.

HIGH RISK: JOHN

John is a 40-year-old executive of a large manufacturing company, who is continually under pressure from work deadlines, does no exercise, is overweight, eats lots of junk foods and has a bad family history of heart disease.

His blood fats profile is:

Cholesterol	7.9	(normal: less than 5.5)
Triglycerides	3.3	(normal: less than 1.7)
HDL	0.7	(normal: greater than 1.1)
LDL	5.7	(normal: less than 3.5)
LDL/HDL	8.1	(normal: less than 3.5)

John has LDL/HDL imbalance. His high levels of LDL put him in the 'at risk of heart disease' category. Note that John also has high triglycerides, which often accompany low HDL levels (see Chapter 21 on the Metabolic Syndrome).

LOW RISK: HELEN

Helen, a 40-year-old woman who regularly runs marathons, is lean, does not smoke, has no family history of heart disease, and has a low-fat, low-cholesterol nutrition program.

Helen's blood fat profile is:

Total cholesterol	4.4
Triglycerides	1.1
HDL	2.4
LDL	1.5
LDL/HDL	0.6

Her HDL/LDL balance scales are tipped in the other direction. In other words, her HDL is high, while her LDL is low. Thus, she has an extremely low risk of heart disease.

You will note that the levels for Helen's HDL are significantly higher than for John. Women often have higher HDL than men—one of the reasons why pre-menopausal women have lower heart attack rates.

INDETERMINATE RISK: JEAN

Some people have high levels of both HDL and LDL cholesterol, and relatively normal LDL/HDL cholesterol ratios. Jean's blood fat profile is:

Total cholesterol	7.0
Triglycerides	1.1
HDL	2.0
LDL	4.5
LDL/HDL	2.2

People with Jean's blood fat profile appear to have a normal risk, as suggested by the ratio. Others have a low risk as suggested by the high HDL, while others have a high risk as suggested by the high LDL levels.

Many cholesterol specialists tend to treat levels of HDL and LDL cholesterol independently and therefore strive to lower LDL further. Jean's profile is not common and may reflect several subgroups, where risk is variable.

In practice, we take particular care with this group to assess whether there is clogging of the arteries (see Chapter 1). In the presence of clogging, we recommend the patient aim to lower his or her LDL levels. HDL and LDL are not the only factors that can influence whether a person is at risk of developing heart disease. For example, a heavy smoker may be at increased risk in spite of a good blood fat profile.

Functions of HDL

In contrast to LDL, HDL has many functions, some of which have only recently been discovered.

For many years, scientists thought that the major role of HDL was to transport cholesterol from tissues back to the liver, thereby completing the cycle of cholesterol movement to and from the liver. This function of HDL was called *reverse cholesterol transport*, and seemed to explain why high HDL levels were associated with low rates of heart disease.

High HDL was associated with relatively large amounts of cholesterol being removed from the tissues back to the liver. In this situation, the arteries were not able to accumulate cholesterol and therefore were less affected by atherosclerosis (see Chapter 1).

Many studies have confirmed the link between less severe atherosclerosis and high HDL levels, indicating that *reverse cholesterol transport* may be important in protecting the arteries from cholesterol accumulation and atherosclerosis. Other functions of HDL are now known to include:

- Preventing oxidation.
- Maintaining the function of the cells lining the blood vessels.
- Acting as a 'storage site' of cholesterol, triglycerides, and phospholipids, which can be transferred to other lipoproteins in the blood.
- Preventing inflammation.

All these actions help our blood vessels to function normally and prevent our arteries from clogging.

The Baddie—LDL

As discussed earlier, cholesterol is an integral part of cell membranes, and can be thought of as a 'building block' for cells. All tissues and cells of the body therefore need cholesterol to function, and all have the capacity to synthesise or 'use' cholesterol.

But nature has evolved a clever way to conserve energy and simplify the body tissues' need for cholesterol by allowing the liver to synthesise most of the body's cholesterol.

The liver is the body's manufacturing site, where after manufacture, cholesterol is packaged, and secreted into the blood in the form of very low-density lipoproteins (VLDL).

In the blood, VLDL is converted into LDL, which then transports cholesterol to the other tissues.

The tissues have a way of capturing any LDL particles that happen to be close enough, by means of *LDL receptors*, which reach out into the blood from the surface membranes like vacuum cleaners.

There are thousands of LDL receptors on the surface of each cell, and when an LDL receptor has trapped an LDL, the receptor folds inwards and forms a little spherical particle within the cell. The LDL receptor-derived particle is then broken down to release cholesterol into the cell.

These steps were worked out in the 1970s in the Texas laboratories of Michael Brown and Joseph Goldstein, who ultimately shared the Nobel Prize in Medicine for their discovery.

How can LDL and HDL be measured?

A fasting blood sample is necessary to accurately measure LDL, because it is calculated from levels of cholesterol, triglycerides and HDL.

Because triglyceride levels are raised after a meal, it is necessary to avoid food and drink (other than water) for 12–14 hours before a blood test.

Example

Tom has his non-fasting blood fat profile measured. His levels are:
- cholesterol   6.5
- triglycerides   4.3
- HDL   1.0
- LDL   3.5
- LDL/HDL   3.5

After an overnight fast, Tom's profile is:
- cholesterol   6.5
- triglycerides   2.2
- HDL   1.0
- LDL   5.0
- LDL/HDL   5.0

Look at the discrepancy between the LDL and LDL/HDL ratios in the two test results. To accurately measure LDL, fasting blood is necessary. These days, direct measurement of LDL in non-fasting blood is possible, but these methods are not routinely used in clinical practice. Note also that Tom's cholesterol and HDL levels were not altered by fasting. This is usually the case (unless triglycerides were very high). Because LDL levels can rapidly fall after heart attack, injury or surgery, measurement must be made either within 24 hours or at least four weeks later.

When should LDL and HDL cholesterol be measured?

All adults aged 18 and above should have at least one initial measurement of their blood fats, including cholesterol, triglycerides, LDL and HDL. 'Know your cholesterol number' was the refrain of a successful education program carried out in recent years in the US. The following people should have blood fat testing because of their increased risk of cardiovascular disease:
- Personal history of vascular disease (including angina, heart attack, stroke, transient ischaemic attack ('mini-stroke'), carotid disease or disease of the arteries of the

legs, pelvis or abdomen.
- Diabetes
- High blood pressure
- Overweight
- Family history of vascular disease
- Cigarette smokers

If blood fats are at acceptable levels, it is recommended that the test is repeated at least every five years. If blood fats show high levels of risk, more frequent testing is carried out (often six-monthly).

What are the recommended levels of LDL and HDL?
Recommended levels depend on whether a person has other coronary risk factors, such as diabetes and previous cardiovascular disease. There is also variation between different countries.

SUMMARY

- Measurement of only cholesterol in the blood is no longer sufficient to determine risk of clogging of the arteries.
- It's also necessary to measure levels of HDL (the 'good' cholesterol) and LDL (the 'bad' cholesterol)
- Once HDL is measured, and LDL calculated, their independent and opposite contributions to risk can be determined and treatment planned accordingly.
- People with high LDL accompanied by low HDL are at particularly increased risk of heart attack and stroke. This is a 'walking time bomb' situation, and urgent treatment is necessary.
- Those with low LDL and high HDL (usually of genetic origin) are at particularly low risk.
- The underlying causes of low and high HDL and LDL need to be investigated and corrected if necessary in any management plan for blood fat control.

10
Blood Fat Levels in Adults and Children

Adults

Finland used to have one of the highest rates of heart disease. Their traditional diet was heavily weighted towards full-cream dairy products. The government intervened with a program of lowering cholesterol-rich food intake and as a result the blood fat levels of the population decreased significantly and so, of course, did the rates of heart disease.

In most populations, there is a close relationship between average blood cholesterol levels and the death rates from heart attack, the steepness of the curve varying between different countries. One of the early studies was the Seven Countries Study, in which there was almost a straight-line relationship between average cholesterol levels and heart attack rates for Japan, Yugoslavia, Greece, Italy, the Netherlands, US and Finland.

Average blood fat levels vary with age

The range of blood fat levels in adults is similar in most Western industrialised countries, and is associated with a relatively high incidence of coronary heart disease. These ranges are:

- Cholesterol: in men the average varies with age from about 5.0 at age 25–34 to 5.5 at age 75 or above. In women the average level varies from 5.0 at age 25–34 to 5.9 at age 75 or above.
- LDL: average levels in men are 3.3–3.5, and for women 2.9–3.6 depending on age.
- Triglycerides: average levels in men are 1.3–1.6, and for women 1.1–1.5 depending on age.
- HDL: average levels in men are 1.2–1.3, and for women 1.5–1.7 depending on age.

Increasing use of medications to lower cholesterol and triglycerides

The use of medications to lower cholesterol and triglycerides has increased from about 1 per cent of men and women in 1980 to 3.3 per cent of women and 5.1 per cent of men in 2000. Use of medication to lower cholesterol and triglycerides is much higher in older age groups, e.g. about 20 per cent of men and women aged 65–74 years.

The treatment gap

Of those not taking medications, three-quarters still have high blood cholesterol or triglyceride levels, suggesting a *treatment gap* of people who should have been receiving treatment but were not.

A high proportion of the population has abnormal blood fat levels, in spite of the use of medications to help control them. The proportions of the population with abnormal blood fats are:

- Cholesterol: 40–70 per cent (highest in older women)
- LDL: 35–60 per cent (highest in older women)
- HDL: 5–20 per cent (highest in men of all ages)
- Triglycerides: 20–30 per cent (similar in men and women)

These results show that we need to pay closer attention to preventing, treating and controlling high cholesterol levels. Many millions of people have high cholesterol levels, as well as abnormal triglycerides, HDL and LDL levels. All these people are at increased cardiovascular risk, and controlling cholesterol and triglyceride levels is one key to prevention of heart attack and stroke.

Children

We tend to think about cholesterol as a problem that occurs in middle life. Many patients tell me they think cholesterol is part of the middle-age spread, something they need not bother about until perhaps their mid-to-late forties.

This, of course, is not really so. Some people are born with high cholesterol and need control from an early age.

In some families, high cholesterol is a genetic disease. Sometimes when adults present with problems, their children as well as their siblings need to be monitored.

Certainly, even in families where cholesterol is not a genetic problem, it is a good idea to raise awareness of the importance of low-fat, low-cholesterol nutrition, plus regular exercise, at an early age. As always, the ounce of prevention is better than the pound of cure!

At birth, levels of cholesterol and other blood fats are very low because nutrients have been provided from the mother via the umbilical cord, rather than from the diet via intestinal absorption. Cholesterol levels are similar for most animal species, including humans, cats, dogs and pigs. Children of varying racial backgrounds have similar levels. Average levels are:

- Cholesterol: 2.0 (range 0.25–6.0)
- Triglycerides: 0.4 (range 0.06–1.25)
- HDL: 0.7 (range 0.1–2.5).
- LDL: 1.1 (range 0.2–4.5)

The variation in each blood fat reflects genetic differences, laboratory variation and effects of the birth process (for example, longer births result in transiently higher cholesterol levels). For these reasons, measuring cholesterol at birth is not a reliable way to detect babies with genetic high cholesterol. At the age of five days, however, when heel-prick blood samples are used to detect other genetic disorders such as low thyroid activity, genetic high cholesterol can be detected reliably.

After birth, blood cholesterol levels gradually increase during the first few months of life to plateau at about 4.2 by age six. This *cholesterol plateau* depends on environmental factors, and varies from country to country. The average levels in Australia and the USA are similar (about 4.2), while those in Mexico and India are much lower (3.0 to 3.5). Finland, a country with a high heart attack rate, used to have the highest average blood cholesterol level of about 6.0 in 8–10 year olds, until measures were taken to lower intake of full-cream daily foods, which has reduced the level significantly.

Upper limits of 4.5 in children and 5.5 in adults have been set for blood cholesterol levels. Children whose blood cholesterol levels are slightly higher than 4.5 tend to have a diet high in cholesterol, saturated fats and sugars, and usually their blood cholesterol levels return to normal once they start eating differently.

Some children have cholesterol levels over 6.0; there is often a genetic cause for this. These children often need drugs to help lower their cholesterol to below 4.5. Most tolerate the drugs well and if the problem is explained properly to them and they are regularly monitored by their doctors, the drug regimen does not impact negatively on their young lives and will help them maintain acceptable levels of cardiovascular health during adulthood.

It is always important to involve parents and even siblings and grandparents, so that the whole family understands the purpose and necessity of continuing the program. Because this is so important, we'll look at genetic disorders of cholesterol in more detail in Chapter 11.

During adolescence, blood HDL levels gradually increase in girls and decrease in boys, so that in young adults, HDL levels are about 0.3 higher in women than in men. The decrease in HDL in boys appears to be related to weight gain and to an effect of male hormones (testosterone). There is also some fluctuation in cholesterol and triglyceride levels during adolescence, possibly related to hormonal as well as dietary factors. Food guidelines are similar to those for adults:

- Reduce total fat and saturated fat intake
- Increase fibre (complex carbohydrate) intake
- Reduce sugar intake
- Alter the intake of dietary fats to allow about equal proportions of polyunsaturated, monounsaturated and saturated fats
- Eat a varied diet

Assessing cardiovascular risk in children is very similar to adults. Some children have high blood cholesterol, LDL and triglyceride levels and low HDL, just as in adults. There are overweight children with high blood pressure, who do relatively little physical activity. Others have diabetes and still others eat a diet high in saturated fats and cholesterol. Some are beginning to smoke cigarettes.

In the light of what we now know medically, it seems appropriate to measure children's risk factors for cardiovascular disease in late primary school or early secondary school. A finger-prick blood sample can be used to measure blood fats.

It is best to start on a program of preventing coronary heart disease at an early age, before lifelong habits are formed. Children are at the ideal age for risk factor screening, assessment and education.

SUMMARY

- There are differences in blood fat levels between men and women at different ages and a significant proportion of the population has unsatisfactory blood fat levels.
- The percentage of women with high LDL levels increases dramatically after the menopause.
- Many men and women who take blood fat-lowering medication do not achieve low enough levels.
- Blood fat levels at birth are low and similar in all races.
- In infancy, nutritional and genetic factors influence blood fat levels. Bad lifestyle habits in childhood put adults at risk of cardiovascular disease.
- Genetic high blood fats can be detected in children.
- Preventive measures may best be undertaken in childhood when lifelong habits are being formed (especially not to smoke cigarettes).

11
High Blood Fats — Acquired or Inherited?

You can be born with the propensity for high blood fat levels (genetic) or you can acquire them during your lifetime through infection, illness, lifestyle or even occupation and where you live.

If you have a diet high in saturated fats and cholesterol-laden foods, allow yourself to become overweight and don't do much physical exercise, it's likely that your levels of blood cholesterol and triglycerides will be far too high.

Genetic causes of high blood fats are relatively uncommon and we'll discuss them later in this chapter.

Acquired causes (that is, problems you acquire after birth, as opposed to genetic causes you inherit at birth) are relatively common, and are due to disturbances in the body's metabolism. Many of these can be diagnosed from the blood sample used for measuring blood fats.

Acquired causes of high blood fats

- Diabetes
- Low thyroid activity
- Kidney diseases (either excessive protein loss in the urine or kidney failure)
- Blockage of bile outflow from the liver
- Anorexia
- Certain disturbances of the immune system
- Pregnancy
- Certain drugs

All of the above conditions, except *diabetes* and *low thyroid activity,* can be picked up by doctors from a patient's history and examination.

Diabetes

Diabetes is a condition in which the person shows a high blood glucose level. There are specific pathological changes in small blood vessels, leading to damage of the kidneys and eyes. Diabetes increases one's risk of heart attack and stroke, as well as arterial disease of the legs.

Diabetes is discussed in detail in Chapter 21. About 7 per cent of the population has this disease, and it is therefore a relatively uncommon cause of high blood cholesterol levels.

Far more common, affecting up to 20 per cent of people, is a pre-diabetic condition called *impaired glucose tolerance*, in which there are no symptoms of diabetes, no evidence of blood vessel pathology, and normal fasting blood glucose levels. After an oral glucose load, however, the blood glucose levels are higher than normal.

People who are overweight, don't do enough exercise, and who eat too much dietary sugar and saturated fats tend to have impaired glucose tolerance. Furthermore, they are often smokers, have high blood pressure, and have high blood cholesterol and triglyceride levels.

These abnormalities, however, can largely be corrected by reducing weight, changing the diet, reducing total fat, sugar and saturated fat intake, and doing more exercise.

Low thyroid activity

Low thyroid activity is an important cause of high blood cholesterol levels because proper replacement treatment with thyroid hormone will lower blood cholesterol levels to normal and significantly improve the patient's wellbeing. Low thyroid activity is a very insidious disease, often occurring over several years. Because the changes are so slow and often unnoticeable, the patient's friends, family and doctor might not even recognise the condition.

People with low thyroid activity are very sensitive to cold, as their metabolism becomes slower than normal and their body temperature also falls slightly. Their skin becomes dry and cracked; their hair becomes fine and brittle and may fall out. Their face becomes puffy and pale. Their pulse rate slows. They may experience heart failure, with shortness of breath and swollen ankles.

Because these changes can take several years to develop, low thyroid activity is sometimes suspected for the first time when the patient is seen by a new doctor while the usual doctor is away, or by a friend or relative whom the patient has not seen for a long time.

People with low thyroid activity may have very high blood cholesterol levels, often up to 12, depending on the severity of the condition. Slightly high blood cholesterol levels of 6–8 occur with slightly low thyroid activity. Most people respond to thyroid hormone tablets which rapidly bring cholesterol levels under control.

Many of the above symptoms, to varying degrees, may also be associated with high triglyceride levels. Uncontrolled diabetes is particularly prone to high triglycerides, which may be more dangerous than high cholesterol because of inflammation of the pancreas (acute pancreatitis) if triglyceride levels are higher than 11.

Nephrotic syndrome

A kidney disorder in which large amounts of protein are lost in the urine.

Kidney failure

People with kidney failure may have a sallow complexion as a result of mild anaemia. Furthermore, their blood chemistry shows high levels of urea and creatinine because the poorly functioning kidneys do not properly remove these substances.

Blockage of bile outflow from the liver

The medical term for this is 'obstructive jaundice'. A deep yellow pigment called bilirubin is normally excreted in the bile. If excretion from the liver is blocked, the accumulating bilirubin causes the whites of the eyes and the skin to turn yellow, the urine to darken, and the bowel motions to lose colour.

Anorexia

This is recognisable in its later stages by extreme weight loss, although in the early stages it may resemble overzealous dieting to reduce weight. Apart from occasional people with severe anorexia who may have very high blood cholesterol levels (up to 14), there are no characteristic changes in blood chemistry.

Disturbances of the immune system

These may cause a wide variety of symptoms, but blood chemistry screening can detect high levels of proteins called *globulins*, which the immune system tends to overproduce.

Pregnancy

Women who are either *pregnant or breastfeeding* should be aware that their blood cholesterol and triglyceride levels may be high because of changes in their hormone levels.

Women who are pregnant or breastfeeding should not take cholesterol-lowering or triglyceride-lowering medications because of potential harm to the baby. But once the baby is born and breastfeeding has ceased, these medications can be resumed safely.

A pregnant woman's diet—both during and after pregnancy—needs to be well balanced with adequate supplies of nutrients and energy, and should be supervised by a health professional.

Drugs

Many drugs can influence blood cholesterol and triglyceride levels. They include steroids, oestrogens, anti-acne drugs, and protease inhibitors for HIV infection. If in doubt about your medication, check with your doctor or pharmacist.

Inherited high blood fats

We have a saying in cardiology: The best thing you can do for your cardiovascular health is to choose your parents carefully.

In other words, genetics has a major effect on our cardiovascular health. I always tell my patients who have heart disease in their families that those who carry a genetic load need to be even more pro-active in their attitudes and sustain an ongoing program for keeping their arteries clear.

For many people, of course, the combination of genetic and environmental factors needs to be assessed.

Studies of populations in different countries have shown blood cholesterol and triglyceride levels are profoundly affected by environmental factors such as eating a diet high in saturated fat and cholesterol, being overweight, and not doing enough physical exercise.

Yet environmental factors do not completely explain the wide variation in cholesterol and triglyceride levels within the normal population. The range of cholesterol varies from less than 3.0 (in about 0.3 per cent of the population) to greater than 9.0 (in about 0.7 per cent of the population). The range for triglycerides varies from about 0.5–1.9. Most people, of course, have cholesterol and triglyceride levels close to the population average (about a third have cholesterol levels between 5.0 and 6.0, and triglyceride levels between 0.9 and 1.5).

There are a number of inherited conditions—with either abnormally high or low blood fat levels—that may increase or reduce the risk of heart attack and stroke, depending on what the condition is. These genetic disorders are also modified by dietary and other environmental influences.

CASE STUDY: STEPHEN

Stephen, a 28-year-old farmer, has a condition called *familial hypercholesterolaemia* (FH). *Familial* refers to any condition that is inherited (i.e. has a genetic basis); *hyper* means high or raised; anaemia means anything to do with the blood. FH therefore means high blood cholesterol of genetic origin. It refers to high cholesterol caused by an abnormal gene for the LDL receptor.

Stephen's father died suddenly at the age of 42, after suffering from chest pain from clogging of the coronary arteries since he was 36. Stephen's paternal grandfather also died suddenly at the age of 49. Stephen's paternal great-grandfather died of a 'heart condition' at 50. Five of Stephen's paternal uncles either died of a heart attack or developed chest pain at an early age. At least one uncle had chest pain in his thirties, and another died of a heart attack aged 41. Stephen's mother is well and almost everyone on his mother's side of the family has been long-lived.

Stephen's family tree is typical of FH—on one side about half the members have had early-onset heart disease, while on the other side most people have normal life expectancies. Half of the children of a person with FH will also have FH, while the other half will be normal. Boys and girls are affected equally. This is the classical Mendelian inheritance pattern of an *autosomal dominant* gene, like the colour of pea flowers as originally studied by Gregor Mendel, the 'father of genetics'.

Before treatment, Stephen's blood cholesterol was 14.6. It is now down to 5.5 with medications. Stephen has the typical features of very high blood cholesterol levels. Cholesterol has been deposited in the outer edge of the cornea, producing in each eye a pale, thin whitish ring called an *arcus senilis* (see Figure 11.1). This white ring can be seen in people over age 60 that have normal cholesterol levels, but in young people it is usually a sign of high blood cholesterol.

Stephen also has cholesterol deposits in the tendons of his hands on the back of each knuckle, visible and felt as small bumps. These are called *tendon xanthomas* (see Figure 11.3).

Figure 11.1 (left) Arcus senilis is a white arc of cholesterol deposited in the outer rim of the cornea.

Figure 11.2 (right) xanthelasmas are cholesterol deposits in the eyelids.

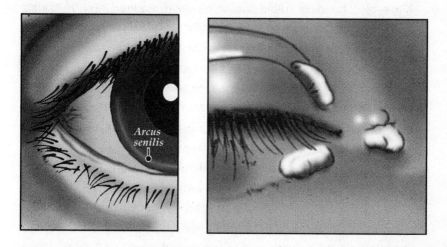

Figure 11.3. Tendon xanthomas are firm bumps in the tendons of the knuckles or in the Achilles tendon at the ankle.

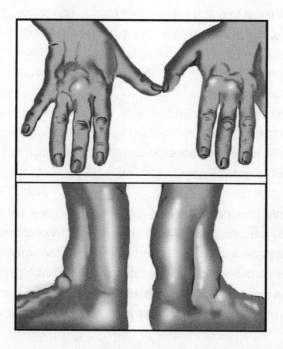

He also has cholesterol deposits in the Achilles' tendons, which are consequently thicker than normal.

Stephen has yellow flat patches on the *surface* of his lower eyelids— cholesterol deposits called *xanthelasmas* (from the Greek *xanthos* = yellow). Xanthelasmas, like arcus senilis, is also sometimes detectable in older people with normal blood cholesterol levels.

For many years, Stephen has been able to maintain normal blood cholesterol levels by taking cholesterol-lowering medications (a statin and resin in maximum doses), and by following a strict cholesterol-lowering diet. His tendon xanthomas and xanthelasmas have decreased in size, but the arcus has remained.

He has no symptoms of clogging of the arteries and is very likely to outlive all his paternal relatives who were affected by FH.

Stephen has two children. Paul, aged seven, also has FH because his cholesterol level is 8.0—about twice normal. Jenny, aged two, does not have FH because her cholesterol level is 2.7 (normal less than 4.5).

Paul has been on the same diet as Stephen, and his cholesterol level has fallen to 6.9. It is likely that Paul will be treated with a statin after ten years of age, in light of recent studies of children with FH:

- Statin treatment in children has been shown to be safe and effective, with normal growth and development while on treatment.
- Clinical trials in children with FH have shown that statin treatment prevents thickening of the carotid arteries.
- In FH-affected children, clogging of the coronary arteries occurs in their teens.

'The earlier the better' seems best when treating FH in children, especially when a parent has had clogging of the coronary arteries at an early age. However, the age at which to start statin treatment is often not clear-cut. Each child must be judged individually according to age, acceptance of blood tests and medications, family history, severity of cholesterol level and wishes of the child and family. In general, children are started on statins once they've reached ten years of age. Studies have shown that most parents are keen to have their children tested for FH if there is the chance they have inherited the condition, and that it can be successfully treated by statin therapy. Lowering the LDL of FH-affected children is now an accepted part of normal medical practice in the hope that it will delay and even prevent clogging of the arteries.

The discovery and investigation of LDL receptors, and the delineation of the underlying metabolic defect in FH, earned Brown and Goldstein the Nobel Prize in 1986. Brown and Goldstein pioneered a method to measure LDL receptor activity in human cells grown in the laboratory. Measurement of low LDL receptor activity is one way to diagnose FH, but the method is available in only very few research laboratories. Brown and Goldstein were able to diagnose FH in an unborn child by removing cells from the amniotic fluid surrounding the developing baby, and by detecting absent LDL receptor activity in the cells.

Hopefully the discoverer of statins (Akiro Endo, who recently won the prestigious Japan Prize for his research) will also win a Nobel Prize, because statins have been of enormous benefit for people with FH as well as other people with high LDL levels.

Why FH is important:
- FH occurs in a significant proportion of adults who suffer from heart attack at a relatively early age.
- FH can be readily diagnosed by measuring blood cholesterol levels both in adulthood and at any age in childhood.
- Effective means of treatment are now available (especially with statin drugs).
- In adults and children who are affected by FH, clogging of the arteries is a lot less severe when treated with cholesterol-lowering drugs.
- Premature heart attack may be prevented by effective and early treatment.

Inherited high triglycerides

The most common form of inherited high triglycerides is familial combined hyperlipidaemia (we'll call it FCHL). This condition is caused by overproduction of triglycerides and apoB in the liver. Some family members have high blood cholesterol levels, others have high blood triglycerides, and others again have both high cholesterol and triglycerides. About one in 200 people have FCHL.

Unlike FH, we cannot detect FCHL in childhood because blood triglyceride levels may not increase above normal until after puberty. FCHL is treated by restricting the patient's intake of sugars and saturated fats. Some people need drugs such as a statin and/or a fibrate. There are rare conditions that are associated with very high triglyceride levels (e.g. over 40). These are due to one of several abnormal genes which prevent the breakdown of triglycerides in the bloodstream. Special tests are required to diagnose them.

Other genetic disorders

Several other genetic disorders can cause high or low cholesterol and/ or triglycerides. One of the most important is low HDL, which is common in people who have premature heart attacks, and is often due to underproduction of the main protein of HDL, apoA-1.

Gene therapy

As a result of molecular biology being applied to medicine, more and more causes of genetic high cholesterol and triglycerides will undoubtedly be diagnosed in the future.

The hope is that one day we will be able to switch genes on and off at will, and modify the body's responses to not only our inherent genetic makeup but also to diseases caused by external agents such as infections.

A novel technique is gene interference, in which people can be given double-stranded RNA (also called 'silencing RNA') that can switch off a target gene. Andrew Fire and Craig Mello, the discoverers of gene silencing, were awarded the 2006 Nobel Prize in Medicine and Physiology. Clinical trials in people with FH have just begun using silencing RNA for apoB, the main protein of LDL. Once-weekly injections in monkeys of apoB-silencing RNA have been shown to lower LDL by about 80 per cent.

SUMMARY

- High blood fats are often associated with dietary or lifestyle habits (such as alcohol excess). A few have a genetic cause. For the remainder, several medical conditions may be responsible and need to be treated.
- It is important to identify the inherited causes of high blood cholesterol because they occur in a significant proportion of people who suffer from premature clogging of the arteries.
- High cholesterol also occurs in children, especially if one of their parents is affected. Treating children with cholesterol-lowering drugs is normal medical practice.
- Many people with inherited high cholesterol are not aware of their disease.
- If you suspect you may have inherited this condition, check your family history.
- Diagnosing the disease is simple—measure the cholesterol level.
- The genetic causes of high blood triglycerides are less strongly associated with premature heart disease than high cholesterol, but are also important.

12
Testing Your Blood Cholesterol Level

Knowing your blood cholesterol and triglyceride levels is as important as knowing your name and your age.

I often say to patients: 'You are as old as your arteries.' Remembering that cardiovascular disease is the biggest cause of preventable death in our community, it stands to reason that if you have clean, unclogged arteries, your arteries are 'young', no matter how old you actually are.

Conversely, it is sadly true that some quite young people have sick, clogged arteries and are at great risk of early death or at least serious disease. So before starting on a cholesterol-lowering program, you should know your blood cholesterol level. At the same time, measure your levels of triglycerides, HDL and LDL so doctors can accurately assess your risk of heart attack. This will help them plan the most appropriate treatment for you. It's a simple procedure:

1. Make an appointment with your doctor.
2. Your doctor may either refer you to a pathology lab, or make an appointment for you at the surgery to have your blood taken.

Pathology labs can only take blood from people who are referred by their doctor, and will report results only to that doctor.

3. Arrive for your blood test after an overnight fast. Twelve hours of fasting are usually sufficient, but some labs prefer 14 hours. During the period of fasting you must not eat or drink anything other than water. Your usual medication should be continued and taken at the usual times. Fasting is necessary to measure blood triglycerides, which otherwise rise after a meal and may remain high for several hours.

4. Blood cholesterol and HDL levels can be measured without fasting, but this does not allow for LDL calculation, which requires measurement of fasting triglycerides. Levels of blood cholesterol and HDL do not usually differ significantly in non-fasting compared with fasting blood.

The procedure for blood sampling is as follows:
- The skin is swabbed with alcohol and allowed to dry.
- A sterile needle is inserted into a small vein just beneath the skin. This is a painless procedure (a sharp pinprick is sometimes felt momentarily as the needle penetrates the skin).
- Once inside the vein, the needle causes no discomfort.
- 5–10 ml of blood is then withdrawn into a sterile plastic syringe; disposable sterile needles and syringes and careful lab procedures ensure safety—there is no danger of being infected by such viruses as AIDS.

In young children and some adults, a fingertip blood sample may be taken instead. The procedure is similar:
- Cleaning the skin
- Gently massaging the blood towards the fingertip
- Pricking the skin with a short sterile lancet
- Some laboratories have special automated machines that make it even easier

- After the skin is punctured, blood drops are then drawn into a capillary tube

After the test, a sterile plastic strip is placed over the puncture site where there may be minor discomfort and possibly bruising for a day or so. You are free to eat and drink. But remember why you came for the blood test, and eat and drink sensibly!

Your blood results will usually be available in the next day or two, when you will have to make another appointment to discuss them with your doctor.

Your results can be used to measure risk for heart disease and stroke (see Chapter 6).

SUMMARY

- Your blood fats are measured after an overnight fast (water only).
- Take your medications at the usual time.
- Cholesterol, triglycerides and HDL levels are measured in the blood sample and your LDL is calculated.
- Your blood fat levels are important indicators of your risk of heart attack risk.
- You need to assess other risk factors as well to get a complete picture of your cardiovascular health.

13
Balancing the Body's Cholesterol

Cholesterol is necessary for the body to function normally. In fact, we could not survive without it. Problems occur when we have too much in our bloodstream. So where does the extra cholesterol come from? Well, it's no longer news to most people that part of the cholesterol build-up in our blood comes from too much of it in our diet. The rest is manufactured by the liver. So cholesterol build-up is a complicated issue. Cholesterol that we absorb from the diet is a major source of our body's cholesterol, and averages about 300–400 mg daily over a wide range from 50–400 mg daily. One egg yolk contains about 250 mg.

The other source of cholesterol is manufactured by the body in the liver, which produces about 1000 mg daily. The liver very carefully adjusts its manufacturing rate so the total amount of cholesterol in the body remains constant.

This means the liver will cut back cholesterol production if there is increased intake, and vice-versa. The body knows that too much cholesterol is bad for it and has mechanisms to get rid of cholesterol and help maintain a balance between dietary intake and loss:

- The liver makes bile, which contains a significant amount of cholesterol (so much so that gallstones in the gallbladder, where bile is stored, may be formed from excessive cholesterol). Most cholesterol in the bile is reabsorbed from the intestine and returned to the liver. A fraction of the cholesterol is lost in the faeces.
- The liver also converts about 900 mg of cholesterol daily into bile salts, which enter the intestine in bile, just like cholesterol made by the liver. Bile salts are important for digestion of fats. Like cholesterol, most of the bile salts are reabsorbed and returned to the liver and a small amount is lost in the faeces.

We lose about 200 mg of cholesterol daily. When we are in good health, cholesterol balance is always maintained, and cholesterol intake is equal to cholesterol loss.

Dietary cholesterol and heart attack

In countries where people's intake of cholesterol is low (below 200 mg per day) the death rate from heart attack is about three times lower than those populations where cholesterol intake is high (above 500 mg per day).

Cholesterol absorption

Cholesterol in food is absorbed from the small intestine by a specific cholesterol-transporting protein. It then becomes incorporated with other food fats into fatty globules called *chylomicrons* (from the Greek *khulos* = juice and *mikros* = small). These enter the lymphatic vessels that pass from the intestines to the blood circulation. We absorb about 200–600 mg of cholesterol daily, depending on our dietary intake and other factors. Up to 40 per cent of cholesterol (up to 1500 mg daily) may be absorbed.

Response to dietary cholesterol

Each person will respond differently to an increase in the amount of cholesterol in their diet. LDL can increase by 10–60 per cent and HDL by 1–10 per cent. People with high blood cholesterol levels generally have the highest rise in LDL. Those with low blood cholesterol levels can usually eat large amounts of cholesterol with little effect on their LDL levels.

Genetic factors

We've known for quite some time that the response to dietary cholesterol varies between animal species. Rabbits, for example, respond with extremely high blood cholesterol levels, and their arteries rapidly become clogged. Studies in monkeys and other non-human primates have shown that there is a genetic component to how species respond to dietary cholesterol. Animals can be bred to have either a large or small increase in blood cholesterol levels with the same cholesterol intake. A similar phenomenon appears to occur in humans.

There is no easy way to predict your own response to dietary cholesterol changes. The only reliable way is to have your blood cholesterol level measured several weeks after changing your cholesterol intake, when the body's metabolism has adjusted to the change.

Foods to watch out for

What are the cholesterol-containing foods to watch out for when reducing dietary cholesterol intake?

- High amounts of cholesterol (over 400 mg cholesterol per 100 g) are found in very few foods: egg yolk, caviar and organ meats (liver, brain, kidneys and sweetbreads).
- All forms of cooking fat derived from animal sources— butter, dripping and lard—have a high cholesterol content (100–200 mg cholesterol per 100 g).
- Moderately high levels of cholesterol (50–100 mg cholesterol per 100 g) occur in whole milk or full-cream dairy products.

- Moderately high levels (50–150 mg per 100 g) of cholesterol occur in red meats. Similar levels occur in shellfish (oysters, lobster, prawns, crayfish and scallops).
- Slightly lower levels of cholesterol occur in white meats (fish, turkey and chicken).
- Low-cholesterol foods include low-fat dairy products— ricotta and cottage cheese, skimmed milk and yoghurt (10–20 mg per 100 g).

Plants (fruit, vegetables and cereal products) contain no cholesterol. However, if you cook plant dishes with oils like butter, you will be adding cholesterol. Palm and coconut oils have a high content of saturated fats, which raise blood LDL levels.

The range of cholesterol in foods is therefore very broad, from one extreme (plants) to the other (egg yolk, brains and offal).

The average cholesterol intake varies from 200–600 mg per day. Major sources are:
- Red meats (30–40 per cent)
- Dairy foods (10–20 per cent)
- Eggs (10–30 per cent)
- Poultry (5–20 per cent)
- Fish (2–10 per cent)
- Seafood (1–5 per cent)
- Fat spreads (3–4 per cent)

Sugar-rich foods (including buns, cakes, biscuits, chocolates and sweet desserts) can provide up to 10 per cent of dietary cholesterol in those with a sweet tooth but usually account for about 3–4 per cent.

Cholesterol intake is generally proportional to protein and total energy intake.

SUMMARY

- High cholesterol foods include egg yolk and offal (brains, liver, and kidneys).
- All forms of flesh—red meat, poultry, fish and seafood— have relatively high levels of cholesterol.
- All forms of whole milk dairy products—cheese, butter, and ice cream—have high cholesterol content.
- Vegetables, cereals and any other plant foods contain *no* cholesterol.
- Red meats, eggs and dairy foods can provide more than two-thirds of a person's dietary cholesterol.
- Dietary cholesterol is *not* an essential food requirement. The body can meet its own cholesterol needs with almost no dietary cholesterol at all. Some other fats, however, are essential. We'll discuss them in further detail in the chapter on dietary fats and cholesterol control.
- Low-fat does not mean no fat—often it means only slightly reduced fat (and cholesterol). Be careful—read the labels.
- Eating foods rich in cholesterol increases the cholesterol content of all blood fats, but some people raise their LDL significantly. For this reason, a cholesterol intake of less than 150–200 mg daily is recommended for those with high LDL levels.
- The composition of fatty acids in the diet has a greater effect on LDL levels than cholesterol intake, as we'll see in the next chapter.

Part III

You Are Your Arteries

This part explains how your lifestyle choices—
what you eat, how much you drink, exercise
and whether or not your smoke—affect your
arteries, and shows you how eating healthily,
moving your body and quitting smoking can all
help to keep those arteries open.

14
Food Fat: The Facts

A few generations ago, exercise was a much more regular part of daily life. Before cars, people walked or rode horses, women carried large bundles of washing from their coppers and pegged them on the lines, children walked to school rather than were driven, almost every family had fruit trees and a vegie patch in their gardens and far more people performed physical labour rather than sat at desks.

Work was more physically demanding and we needed more nutrition. Our dietary traditions came from Europe, and were based on a high intake of full-cream dairy produce, meat and eggs. You only have to look at the traditional Christmas dinner, which is really just a glamourised version of the weekly Sunday roast dinner, to see the amount of fat in the meat, the gravy, all over the vegetables and in the sugary-fatty pudding, to say nothing of the custards and white sauce.

This kind of eating originates in cold countries, and from a time when people expended lots of energy in their daily lives. It certainly does not suit today's lifestyles.

Modern lifestyles are no longer suited to the old *haute cuisine* of France and much of the rest of Europe.

As we all know, controlling the type and amount of fat in our diet greatly influences not only our cholesterol level, but also our body weight. More about this in Chapter 20.

We learned in Chapter 8 that the visible fats in foods are made of triglycerides. These are from plant sources, such as olive and sunflower oil, and animal sources such as butter and meat.

Almost 30 years ago, it was found that two dietary factors had major effects on changing blood cholesterol levels:

- The amount of cholesterol in the diet.
- The relative proportion of dietary polyunsaturated to saturated fatty acids (P:S ratio). The average diet has a low P:S ratio of about 0.4.

Saturated, polyunsaturated and monounsaturated fatty acids

We also learnt in Chapter 8 that triglycerides are made up of three main sorts of fats: saturated fatty acids, polyunsaturated fatty acids and monounsaturated fatty acids. These differ in structure, shape, and how they are metabolised in the body.

Saturated fatty acids

These are found in:

- Dairy products (butter, cheese, cream, full-cream milk, yoghurt)
- Meats of all kinds (chicken, lamb, beef, pork and veal)
- Chocolates, crisps, coconut oil and palm oil and products containing them (commercial pastries, cakes, biscuits and confections)

We also know that saturated fats in the diet have a powerful effect on increasing LDL levels. On average, for every 1 per cent increase of total energy as saturated fats, a 2 per cent increase in LDL levels occurred.

Polyunsaturated fatty acids

These are found in:

- Vegetable oils such as corn, safflower, soy and sunflower
- Many other oils of plant origin

It's also worth knowing that polyunsaturated fats decrease LDL levels. On average, for every percentage increase of total energy as polyunsaturated fats, there is a 1 per cent decrease in LDL levels.

Two polyunsaturated fats are important because our bodies can't produce them, so we need them in our diet. They are called the essential fatty acids (EFAs) and include linoleic and linolenic acid. The minimum required in adults appears to be 1–2 per cent of total energy intake. Infants who don't have enough EFAs may get dry, scaly skin and irritation where there is folded skin, for example, in the groin and in the folds of the buttocks.

Adults can also get dry scaly skin due to an EFA deficiency, particularly during long-term intravenous nutrition in cases where people can't take their food by mouth.

A daily intake of EFAs equivalent to about 10 ml of corn oil is enough to prevent EFA deficiency. This is readily provided by a usual cholesterol-lowering diet in which 10–20 per cent of calories come from fat, and the P:S ratio is 1.0 or more.

Monounsaturated fats

These are found in olive oil, canola (rapeseed) oil, nuts and avocados, and also in significant proportions in some cooking fats, polyunsaturated oils, milk and dairy products, and meats of all kinds, including red and white meat and fish. If we were to replace dietary saturated fats with monounsaturated fats, polyunsaturated fats or carbohydrates, LDL levels would fall by about the same amount.

Other fats

These include omega-3 fatty acids (omega-3s) and trans-saturated fatty acids.

Omega-3s

Omega-3s mainly occur in seafood; our bodies cannot produce them. They are polyunsaturated fats with a different structure from the usual polyunsaturated fats of plants.

Omega-3s are synthesised by very simple organisms at the origin of the marine food chain: algae and plankton. These small organisms are eaten by larger organisms, and the process continues as larger fish eat smaller fish. The end result is that fish oil may contain more than 50 per cent of total fatty acids as omega-3s.

In plant-derived foods, there are significant amounts of another type of omega-3 called alpha-linolenic acid (ALA). It is found in fruit, vegetables, nuts (especially walnuts), canola oil (10 per cent ALA), linseed oil (50–60 per cent ALA), mustard oil and soybean oil. One study has shown a lower heart attack rate in people who added fruit, nuts and vegetables or mustard and soybean oils to a low-fat diet.

We will discuss omega-3s in more detail in Chapter 15.

Trans-saturated fats

Trans-saturated fats are found naturally in animal fats, butter, shortening, and in some margarine through hydrogenation of polyunsaturated fats during the manufacturing process. They increase LDL, reduce HDL, and have been shown to increase the risk of heart attack.

Getting the right balance

For most people, changing the nature of dietary fats is more important than cutting back on total fat intake.

Many of us have a high fat intake (40 per cent of total energy), with a low P:S ratio of 0.4. Saturated fats supply about half of the total fat intake, polyunsaturates 12–14 per cent, and monounsaturates the rest.

The ideal foods are low in total energy from fat, low in cholesterol and have a balanced ratio of saturates, polyunsaturates and monounsaturates, with a P:S ratio of about 1:1. No single food can meet all these requirements. The meat coming closest in fat composition is turkey without the skin, which has equal proportions of the three fatty acids.

Turkey meat, however, has moderate cholesterol content (50–80 mg/100 g), although it's lower than red meat.

We need about 20–25 g of fat daily. Ideally, we should get this from cereals, fruit, vegetables, low-fat dairy products, legumes, nuts, lean meat, fish, and suitable oils. These foods also reduce the intake of cholesterol and total fat. Compared with a typical Western diet, you can expect a reduction of about 10 per cent in LDL if you adopt this way of eating.

If you need to lose weight, you may need to restrict your fat intake because fats have twice the energy of sugars and proteins.

Read the labels

Nutrition information is usually listed as a table on food packaging or wrapping. Average serving sizes are used in the tables (note: serving sizes are becoming larger and are partly to blame for the epidemic of overweight in modern society).

Many low-fat products contain a lot of sugar. Low-sugar varieties may also be available. If there is no label, the ingredients are listed in descending order of weight. If fat is one of the first three ingredients, the food is probably high in fat.

Suitable or less suitable? Table 14.1 gives a guide.

Making the right choices

If you are among the 50 per cent of adults with cholesterol levels above 5.5, it is very important that you reduce your intake of whole-fat dairy products, egg yolks, red meats and visible fats. You should also reduce your intake of saturated fats.

All food items now have the content of saturated and total fats printed on the packaging. It's simple—read the labels!

Table 14.1. Suitable and less suitable foods.

Food	Suitable	Less suitable
Fruit	All	None

Cereal	Most	Toasted muesli
Bread	Most	Croissants, Danish pastry, brioche
Spreads	Mono- or poly-unsaturated with less than 0.9 per cent trans-fatty acids	Butter, butter blends, margarines with more than 0.9 trans-fatty acids
Milk	Skim (0.1 per cent fat)	Full-cream
Yoghurt	Low fat	Natural
Sandwich filling	Salad vegetables, canned fish, lean meat, cottage or ricotta cheese, avocado	Salami, liverwurst, pate, processed delicatessen meats
Dressings	Vinaigrette	Creamy, egg-based mayonnaise
Crackers	Ryvita, Cruskit	All others
Soups	Low fat	Other
Meat, fish, poultry	Lean	Battered, fried, crumbed, pastried
Snacks	Nuts, fruit, bread, low-fat crackers	Crisps, chips, most savoury snacks, biscuits

Limiting intake of saturates and trans–saturates

- Limit intake of full-fat dairy foods.
- Avoid visible fat in or on the surface of meat by purchasing lean meat and trimming away visible fat.
- Avoid take-away, fried and commercially baked foods (unless they are prepared from unsaturated oils).
- Avoid coconut and palm oils and products made from them (commercial pastries, biscuits, cakes and confections, or products including vegetable oil).
- Use low-fat dairy products.
- Avoid butter—use unsaturated margarine spreads instead.
- Use margarines containing a stated content of less than 0.9 per cent trans-fats.

- Limit cheese and ice-cream to twice a week or less.
- Limit fatty meats (sausages and delicatessen meats such as salami). Use lean ham, chicken, fish or roast meats.

Increasing intake of polyunsaturates and monounsaturates
- Use a variety of plant oils (olive, canola, peanut, safflower, corn, sunflower, macadamia, grape seed, soybean).
- Use suitable margarines.
- Eat nuts and grains.
- Use salad dressings and mayonnaise made from these oils.
- Soy drinks with added calcium can replace low-fat milk.
- Use various olive oils such as light, virgin, extra-virgin or cold-pressed; all have a suitable fatty acid composition.

Reducing total fat and cholesterol
- Limit egg yolks, full-cream products, meat and offal.

Increasing omega-3s
- Eat at least two fish meals a week (fresh or canned).
- Increase the intake of plant omega-3s through fruit, vegetables, soy and nuts.

Snacking wisely
- For snacks, eat unsalted plain nuts, fresh fruit and other snacks (see Part VII: Low-Chol Cuisine).
- Use legumes (peas, beans or lentils), vegetables and grain-based foods (bread, pasta, rice and noodles) as the primary basis for meals, with added meats as the secondary ingredient as in some kinds of Asian cooking. Legumes include dried peas, chickpeas, soybeans, black-eyed beans, Lima beans, cannelli beans and others.
- An easy way to choose vegetables is to select a variety of colours—red, orange, yellow, green and white.

Taking it away

- Suitable take-away foods are those with vegetables, noodles, rice, pasta and vegetable-based sauces.
- Avoid pastries, pies, sausage rolls, crisps, cheese-based pizzas, hamburgers and creamy pastas.

SUMMARY

- Be aware of the kinds of fat we are eating, as well as the quantity. 'Fat makes fat' refers to the high energy content of fatty foods (about twice that of carbs and protein), and the tendency to put on weight easily when we eat too much of them. Fat, however, can also be 'bad' (high saturated fat content) or 'good' (high monounsaturated and omega-3 content).
- Most of us need to reduce the amount of saturated fats in our diets, by changing to low-fat dairy products, and limiting our consumption of cheese, eggs and meat.
- Eating fish is recommended as a source of low fat, high-quality protein containing lots of 'good' omega-3s, with a moderate cholesterol content.
- Read the labels when buying food—choose low saturated fat, low sugar, and low cholesterol products. Treat your home—that is your body—as a castle surrounded by a moat. Only let the drawbridge up if the food coming in meets your low-fat, low-cholesterol criteria. Control what comes in and control temptation—no storing away in our cupboards the treats for a 'special' occasion. It is best not to invite them in from the start.

15
Something Fishy

Did your grandmother try to give you a spoonful of cod liver oil when you were little and either ill or recuperating from an illness?

It was possibly the most unpopular health supplement of the 1940s and beyond, when children lacking in ideal nutrition due to war shortages were given a boost with good old-fashioned cod liver oil. How they hated it—and who can blame them?

But grandma and the government knew what they were doing. Fish oils are actually very good for you.

Greenland Eskimos, for example, are an exception to the general rule that a high-fat diet is bad for you. Their diets contain a lot of cholesterol and fat, derived mainly from fish, walrus, seal, polar bear and whale blubber. In spite of this, they have a very low rate of heart attacks, low blood cholesterol, high HDL, and very low levels of triglycerides. They also have a tendency to bleed easily from minor cuts. Fish, seal and whale blubber as well as Eskimo blood are rich in omega-3 fatty acids. Eskimo platelets (the cells involved in blood clotting) are also less sticky than normal, causing Eskimos to bleed for a longer time.

Prostaglandins and platelets

These findings are related to a class of chemical compounds called *prostaglandins*, which are products of the essential polyunsaturated fats we have discussed in Chapter 14.

The protective effects of omega-3s

The anti-platelet action of omega-3s should theoretically inhibit clogging of the arteries. Scientists found evidence to support this when monkeys were fed a high cholesterol diet with and without added fish oils for a 12-month period. The monkeys fed fish oils had 50 per cent less severe clogging of the arteries.

A 20-year study of Dutch townspeople also showed that an average of two fish meals a week (30 g of fish daily) reduced the rate of heart attacks by 50 per cent compared with those not eating fish. Heart attacks were two-thirds lower in those regularly eating 3–4 fish meals per week (36 g of fish daily).

Other studies of different populations have also shown that fish oils help prevent heart attacks. For example, people in China, the US and Europe who ate fish more than once a month on average had a 15 per cent lower rate of fatal heart attack compared with non–fish eaters. There are several reasons for the protective effect of fish oils:

- Fish oils may protect against sudden death by improving the electrical stability of the heart.
- The anti-clotting effect on platelets may prevent blockage of a ruptured coronary artery.
- Damage to the lining of the arteries may be reduced.
- Omega-3s may lower triglycerides and increase HDL levels.
- Fish oils may stabilise plaques. People needing surgery to remove plaques in their carotid arteries were fed fish oils for several weeks before surgery. When the removed plaques were examined under the microscope, they were found to have less inflammation and thicker fibrous caps, suggesting they were more stable.

It should be noted that fish eaters also differ from non–fish eaters because they are generally leaner, exercise more and smoke less. may contribute to the protective effect of fish oils.

Omega-3s in fish

- Most fish contains about 230 mg/100 g of omega-3s, and significant amounts are also found in other seafood: oysters (150 mg/100 g), prawns (130 mg/100 g) and lobsters (105 mg/100 g). The biologically active omega-3s are eicosapentaenoic acid (EPA) and docosahexaenoic acid (DHA). Omega-3s account for up to 92 per cent of the polyunsaturated fats in fish.

Table 15.1. Amount of total fat (per cent weight), EPA, DHA and cholesterol in seafood (mg/100 g wet weight of seafood).

Seafood	Total fat (%)	EPA	DHA	Cholesterol
Abalone	1.0	40	1	131
Aust bass	1.5	37	157	27
Balmain bug	0.7	49	44	44
Bream	0.8	21	123	24
Calamari	1.6	85	192	230
Crab (sand)	0.8	126	94	30
Garfish	1.0	16	106	45
Jewfish	0.6	9	44	33
Mulloway	0.6	17	72	22
Prawn	0.9	59	45	85
Snapper	0.5	5	72	21
Trevally (big eye)	4.7	185	375	32
Tuna (slender)	16.5	965	2199	59
Whiting	0.7 per cent	43	115	33

Eating fish is recommended because fish meat has a moderate cholesterol content (about 60 mg/100 g), is low in fat (usually 1–2 per cent), has a P:S ratio of about 1.4, and contains a high proportion of omega-3s. Fish meat is also low in carbohydrates and high in protein (15 to 25 per cent).

Effects on triglycerides

Omega-3s have been found to reduce blood levels of triglycerides because they inhibit production by the liver. Larger amounts of omega-3s are more effective, and higher levels of triglycerides respond better than lower levels. Omega-3s are therefore very useful for treating high blood triglycerides, especially in combination with other drugs such as statins or fibrates. Fish oils can also be taken in the form of capsules, which contain about 180 mg of EPA and 120 mg of DHA. Two fish meals a week (30–40 grams) is equivalent to about seven capsules of fish oils daily.

Effects on LDL

LDL levels can be increased slightly with omega-3s, especially in those with normal triglycerides.

Effects on HDL

Significantly higher HDL (5–15 per cent) can result from omega-3s, especially when triglyceride levels are high.

Effects on arthritis and inflammation

Because of their effects on prostaglandins, omega-3s also partially suppress the inflammatory response to injury and may also have an effect on suppressing certain functions of the immune system. They have been useful for treating arthritis, asthma and pre-menstrual symptoms.

Plant-derived omega-3s

The most abundant natural sources of omega-3s include fish, shellfish and other marine sources of fat. Terrestrial plants also make omega-3s of a shorter chain length, of which alpha-linolenic acid (ALA) is the most abundant. ALA occurs abundantly in linseed oil (50 per cent), walnut oil (11 per cent) and soybean oil (7 per cent). The National Heart Foundation of Australia recommends a daily intake of at least 2 grams of plant omega-3s (predominantly ALA) because the beneficial effects of plant omega-3s may supplement those of fish oils.

Cod liver oil

Cod liver oil is a rich source of readily available omega-3s, and was a useful supplement to the diet in the war years when dairy food was limited. Taking cod liver oil for prolonged periods can be dangerous, however, because of its high content of vitamins A and D, which we store in the liver. Vitamin D in particular is toxic if consumed in excessive amounts. 20 ml of cod liver oil daily provides about four times the recommended daily allowance for both vitamin A and vitamin D, and toxic symptoms may occur with five times the allowance of vitamin D.

Because levels of vitamins A and D in fish flesh are much lower than in cod liver oil, eating fish regularly is safe.

Taking precautions with fish oils

- **Bleeding:** Omega-3s must be used with caution by anyone taking blood thinners (such as aspirin, clopidogrel, dipyridamole and warfarin). Excessive bleeding may result with a very slight risk of stroke from cerebral haemorrhage.
- **Mercury content:** Long-lived fish that are at the top of the food chain (including marlin, swordfish, broadbill, barramundi and shark) may accumulate more mercury than other species. Pregnant women and children up to six years of age should avoid them because of a slight risk of increased amounts of mercury that may have subtle effects on the brain. These fish should be eaten no more than once a fortnight by pregnant women and young

children, with no other fish eaten. Other fish can be eaten safely (for example a 95 g can of tuna daily). Canned fish may be lower in mercury content than fresh fish because fish used for canning are generally smaller and younger. Other people should eat two or three serves of other fish a week. See www.foodstandards.gov.au for further details.

- **Weight gain:** Weight may increase with large quantities of fish oils. Like any dietary fats, they are high in energy.
- **Rise in blood sugar levels:** Some, but not all, studies have shown a rise in blood sugar levels and deterioration in diabetic control with omega-3 supplements. Diabetics who take fish oils should carefully monitor their glucose levels.
- **Digestive problems:** Larger doses of fish oils may cause nausea and mild stomach and intestinal symptoms, especially 'fishy burps'. Special coated fish oil preparations are available to prevent this symptom.

SUMMARY

- Most experts recommend at least two fish meals a week in preference to fish oil capsules. Two or three meals per week will increase omega-3 intake from about 0.2 g per day (the average for most adults) to 4.8 g per day, providing 1–2 per cent of total energy requirements.
- There is still no evidence that omega-3s are essential fats for humans. Levels of omega-3s are low in committed vegetarians but there don't appear to be any side effects of this. At present, we don't know of any body disturbances in humans as a result of omega-3 deficiency.
- The recognised benefits of omega-3s have led to a great increase in fish consumption around the world.

16
Health
Supplements

Taking 'health' supplements has become increasingly popular. There is always new information on how this herb will prevent that ailment, or how that vitamin mixture is good for some health issue.

Some of my patients seem to positively rattle with pills and potions that they self-prescribe from their local health-food stores.

When my patients come to me for the first time, they complete a questionnaire about their medical history, family history, smoking and alcohol habits, exercise, diet, etc. One question asks: 'Are you taking any non-prescribed medications (vitamins, minerals or other supplements)?'

It seems about half are taking some kind of supplement—usually calcium among older women but commonly vitamins of various kinds among younger men and women.

This 50 per cent response rate indicates that the habit of taking supplements is widespread in our community, as it is in other Western countries. In fact, alternative medicine in the form of herbs and naturopathic substances has become very popular. The size of this market is enormous—in the US, over $US 350 million each year is spent on six herbal supplements alone: ginkgo, echinacea, garlic, ginseng, saw palmetto and St John's wort. Total herbal medicine sales in the US are well over $US 4 billion annually, and a survey of 2000 people found that about 40 per cent were regularly using alternative medicines.

One reason for taking alternative medicines is a common belief that they help lower cholesterol, as promoted in enthusiastic marketing and personal endorsements. Is there scientific evidence for this?

Let's look at the results of some trials to see how effective these supplements are.

These trials randomly divide their subjects into two groups (a computer is used in order to minimise bias between them). The first group (the *treatment* group) is given an active tablet, containing whatever we are testing to see if it has an effect. The second group (the *control* or *placebo* group) is given a tablet with an identical appearance to the treatment group, but this tablet is known to have no effect. The nature of the tablet used by a given subject is blinded to both the doctor and the subject—this is called a *double-blind* study. A double-blind, randomised, placebo-controlled study is therefore one of the most scientifically rigorous designs in medicine, and has become the standard for investigating the effects of almost all new medicines.

Garlic

Sixteen trials of garlic in over 800 people showed on average a very small (4–6 per cent) reduction in cholesterol levels. This compares with the 25–55 per cent achieved with statins (see Chapter 29). Garlic had no effect on levels of LDL and HDL, but triglycerides were reduced significantly.

The largest trial with 900 mg/day of garlic showed no effect in over 100 subjects. Three overall analyses of the effects of garlic have come to different conclusions. Some of the variation in results may reflect differences in the garlic preparations and amounts of the active

113

ingredients (which remain unknown). We can conclude from these results that garlic has a very small effect on lowering cholesterol. We can lower cholesterol more effectively simply by cutting back on saturated fats and cholesterol in the diet (see Chapter 14).

Artichoke

In Europe, people take artichoke to increase secretion of bile by the liver and to lower cholesterol. Small effects on lowering cholesterol and triglycerides were shown in two trials; HDL and triglycerides were unchanged. The studies used about 1.8 g/day of artichoke for 6–12 weeks.

Psyllium and beta-glucan

Psyllium and beta-glucan are soluble plant fibres that had a small effect of lowering cholesterol by 2 per cent in eight trials of over 600 people. The dose of soluble fibre was 8–10g daily for 8–26 weeks. There were no effects on HDL or triglycerides. LDL was reduced slightly. This effect on cholesterol was sufficient for the US Food and Drug Administration (FDA) to approve cholesterol-lowering claims for psyllium (1.8 g four times a day) and beta-glucan (0.75 g four times a day).

Oats

In 25 trials of over 1600 people with average baseline cholesterol of 6.3, oats (equivalent to 15–125g daily of oat bran or 28–170g daily of oatmeal) lowered cholesterol by an insignificant amount—only 0.04. There were no changes in HDL or triglycerides.

Guar gum

This was similar to oats and lowered cholesterol by 0.03, with no effect on triglycerides or HDL. Over 350 people were studied in 18 trials, using 17.5g daily of guar gum for 2–24 weeks.

Chitosan

This is a powder made by grinding up the shells of shellfish, which is said to absorb fats and lower cholesterol levels. There have been four trials of over 300 people, with baseline cholesterol levels between 5.5 and 8. In doses of 0.5–2.4g daily for 4–8 weeks, chitosan lowered cholesterol by 0.2 to 1.1, LDL by 1 to 1.1, triglycerides by 0.3 to 0.9, and raised HDL by 0.04 to 0.1.

Wax alcohols including policosanol

Policosanol is a mixture of long-chain alcohols derived from cane sugar wax. Trials mainly conducted in Cuba, Russia and South America have shown significant lowering of cholesterol and LDL levels in doses of 10 mg and 20 mg daily. Beeswax is another source for wax alcohols and is used to improve athletic performance; however, there is not much scientific evidence to show that it is effective.

Cholesterol experts have been disappointed with policosanol 10 mg daily because little or no cholesterol lowering is usually seen. Experience with policosanol 20 mg daily is limited.

Soy

Small changes in cholesterol levels have been shown in several poorly controlled studies of soy supplements, with 2–5 per cent lowering observed (0.1–0.25). Claims of larger lowering (up to 13 per cent) have been made but these were not scientifically adequate trials. In spite of this, a cholesterol-lowering claim for soy has been approved by the FDA and the UK Health Claims Committee.

Plant sterols

Because of their obvious effects, plant sterols have achieved the status of drugs to lower cholesterol and are discussed in Chapter 31.

Omega-3 fatty acids including fish oils

Omega-3 fatty acids improve blood HDL and triglyceride levels as discussed in Chapter 15.

Other supplements

Single trials have been conducted with aloe vera, red clover, coenzyme Q10, red yeast rice, flaxseed and several other substances but the results need to be confirmed in other studies.

Lecithin

Lecithin is widely believed to 'dissolve' cholesterol when taken as a food supplement in the form of granules or liquid formulae.

Lecithin is a phospholipid, widely found in all plant and animal tissues. The lecithin in many plants has a high proportion of polyunsaturated fatty acids, for example, soybean lecithin from which many commercially available preparations of lecithin are made.

Taking lecithin by mouth is equivalent to taking polyunsaturated fats. There is an increase in dietary P:S ratio and a fall in LDL and cholesterol levels. The same is not true, however, for intravenous lecithin. This has been widely used in Europe, and there are anecdotal reports of improvement in angina and cholesterol levels. Experiments in which cholesterol-fed animals were given intravenous lecithin showed significant improvement in clogging of the arteries, even while cholesterol feeding was continued.

Vitamin C

Vitamin C (ascorbic acid) is probably the most widely taken vitamin supplement. Its use was popularised by the dual Nobel Prize winner Linus Pauling, who recommended it for preventing and treating the common cold. Vitamin C has been reported in some studies to lower blood cholesterol levels and raise HDL levels, while other studies have failed to show any significant changes. It is of no proven benefit in preventing heart attacks.

Vitamin E

Vitamin E, a fat-soluble vitamin stored in the liver and fatty tissues, is the body's natural antioxidant, and plays an important role in maintaining the normal structure of polyunsaturated fats by preventing their oxidation. Vitamin E is transported in the blood within LDL particles, and may also protect LDL from damage by harmful substances derived from oxygen (such as free radicals).

Vitamin E supplements, like lecithin supplements, are widely believed to 'dissolve' cholesterol, but there is no evidence of this.

Vitamin E's chemical name is *alpha-tocopherol*. The daily vitamin E requirement for normal people depends on the amount of dietary polyunsaturated fat; higher vitamin E intake is required for higher polyunsaturated fat intake. About 10 mg of alpha-tocopherol are required daily for the average dietary P:S ratios of 0.4:1. Higher intakes of up to 30 mg/day should be taken with dietary P:S ratios above 1:1.

Vitamin E occurs naturally in plant oils such as wheat germ oil. The richest dietary sources of vitamin E are vegetable oils. Dietary sources of vitamin E content in mg/100 g of various oils are: wheat germ 190, soybean 87, corn 66, safflower 49, sunflower 27, peanut 22 and olive oil 5. Vitamin E is also found in cereals, leafy vegetables, fish, meat, milk and eggs (0.5–5 mg/100 g).

Vitamin E doesn't protect against cardiovascular disease

When blood levels of vitamin E were studied in different populations, high levels were associated with lower heart attack rates. Vitamin E was therefore thought to be 'protective' through its action as an anti-oxidant. Several clinical trials were then performed to test the theory that vitamin E supplements may protect from heart attacks. The results, however, have been negative.

Vitamin E supplements may improve symptoms in some people with clogging of the arteries to the legs. This may be related to reduction in the clotting tendency of the blood with doses of 300–400 mg/day.

Vegetarianism

Vegetarians either avoid animal products completely (true vegetarians or vegans) or allow some form of animal products such as milk and other dairy products, eggs, fish or poultry.

Vegetarians are often health-conscious in other areas; for example, they tend to be non-smokers and to have a relatively low alcohol intake. They often take vitamin supplements—however, vitamin B12 alone may be required because this vitamin is found only in animal products and in small quantities in seaweeds and mushrooms.

The truth of the matter

Why are alternative medicines taken when there is little or no scientific proof of benefit? There are several reasons for this.

- Extensive marketing campaigns make persuasive, largely unsubstantiated and extravagant claims for their products. Often 'feeling better' is the basis for these claims—which may be a placebo effect in any case.
- 'Natural' is a word many use when they give reasons for their choice of alternative medicines. They are convinced that a natural product is safer than one synthesised in the laboratory. But there is little scientific support for this belief.
- People feel more in control of their own health because they are the ones making the decisions—they are therefore 'empowered'.
- Others have experienced side effects to standard medical drug therapy and wish to try alternatives.

The positive results of some alternative therapies in some people may be explained by lifestyle changes (such as changing dietary fats, weight loss and exercise) rather than by the therapy itself.

But we shouldn't deny the possibility that some people respond well to alternative therapies. A great deal of research is being done on naturally occurring substances (anti-cancer drugs in particular). In fact, the first statins were synthesised by fungi.

While there is currently no scientific evidence showing any benefit for heart attack and stroke from taking vitamin or mineral supplements, this is not to say that benefits will not become clear in the future.

The science of nutrition is very young, as is the era of widespread vitamin supplement usage by healthy adults, who are not deficient in any of the vitamins they take as supplements. Further research is needed to determine long-term side effects and benefits of vitamin supplementation, especially in doses that are several hundred times higher than are required for normal body function.

SUMMARY

- Many dietary supplements can affect cholesterol levels, albeit to a small degree.
- Clinical trials of these substances have involved relatively small numbers of people for relatively short periods, using different doses of various preparations. This may be one reason why the overall results are not convincing, but they do need to be compared with the far more convincing results of changes in dietary fats and the use of drugs to lower cholesterol.
- Most experts do not recommend any dietary supplements other than plant sterols.
- For further information on dietary supplements there is a lot of data on the internet, much of which is of questionable scientific validity. One site for information on alternative and complementary medicine is: www.ex.ac.uk/FACT.
- Healthy adults who are eating a balanced diet from a variety of sources do not need vitamin supplements.
- As for all dietary recommendations: no hard-and-fast, inviolable rules can be laid down that will suit everybody. We can only give general guidelines, and it is up to the individual to make the choice.

17
The Effects of Alcohol

I was born in South Australia, where many of Australia's famous wines are grown, so it's no surprise that after a busy day's work, I enjoy sitting on the front veranda facing the setting sun, enjoying an hors d'oeuvre or antipasto accompanied by a glass of chilled white wine—the heavenly drop. The day's stresses and strains evaporate, the light takes on a golden glow, and all is well with the world.

Alcohol, whether white or red wine, an aperitif, champagne, beer or spirits, lends the day a little extra, especially combined with good food and pleasant company.

My wife often says our marriage is glued together by a daily glass of wine! Literature abounds with such anecdotes, and art illustrates them for more of our enjoyment.

One standard drink contains 10g of alcohol (see Figure 17.1). This is the amount in two large glasses (285ml or 10oz) of light beer, one glass of normal beer, one glass (120ml) of wine, one shot (30ml or 1oz) of spirits, and one glass (60ml or 2oz) of fortified wine such as port.

You can now calculate your daily alcohol intake. For example, if you drink two double scotches and two glasses of light beer, that's equivalent to 50g of alcohol (five standard drinks).

Figure 17.1. Alcohol content of different beverages.

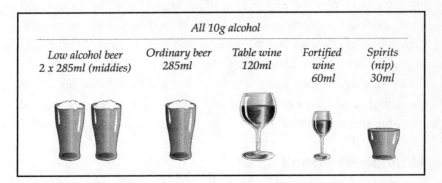

All 10g alcohol				
Low alcohol beer 2 x 285ml (middies)	Ordinary beer 285ml	Table wine 120ml	Fortified wine 60ml	Spirits (nip) 30ml

Alcohol—the bad news

But there is another side to alcohol consumption—also well-documented in art and literature. Science tells us about some harmful effects of heavy alcohol consumption. Like cigarette smoking, alcohol is one of the leading causes of preventable death in industrialised countries. Chronic liver disease (cirrhosis) caused by direct alcohol toxicity is among the leading causes of death. Alcohol is implicated in 50 per cent of fatal traffic accidents, is a major cause of death in young adults, as well as other accidents at home.

The social implications of excessive alcohol consumption are enormous, and include suicides, homicide and robberies. There is an increased risk of cancer of the liver, stomach and pancreas in alcohol drinkers compared with non-drinkers. Some studies have shown alcohol to be implicated in 25 per cent of general hospital admissions and 50 per cent of psychiatric admissions. More than six drinks of alcohol per day during pregnancy may cause harmful physical effects on babies, including possible mental retardation.

Heavy alcohol consumption also increases the risk of heart attack. Heavy drinkers have higher blood pressures and are more often overweight. Alcohol is metabolised in the liver, where increased production of triglycerides may lead to high blood cholesterol and triglycerides. The combination of high blood pressure, overweight, high blood cholesterol and triglycerides as well as cigarette smoking in many cases leads to clogging of the arteries.

The death rate from heart attack has been shown to be up to 3.5 times higher in heavy drinkers than in non-drinkers. Heavy alcohol consumption is therefore a major health problem.

Alcohol—the good news

The evidence has shown, however, that light alcohol consumption is protective for heart attack. The Framingham study showed that alcohol consumption in men aged 50 to 62 was inversely related to the risk of heart attack. This applies to wine, beer and liquor—the alcohol content itself seems to be protective.

One reason for this may be increased blood HDL levels in mild alcohol drinkers. One study has shown each alcoholic drink consumed per day may increase blood HDL levels by about 0.026 in both men and women. This relationship was independent of dietary fat and cholesterol intake and appeared to be due to a direct effect of alcohol on the body. Other factors may also partly account for the protective effects of alcohol. Moderate drinkers (2.5–5 standard drinks per day) eat less cholesterol and dietary fat than either non-drinkers or heavy drinkers (five or more standard drinks per day).

Another reason for a protective effect of alcohol is that certain components, especially in red wine, may act as anti-oxidants. These protect LDL from damage by products of oxygen such as free radicals. The antioxidants in wine are called *flavonoids*, and are extracted from the grape skins during fermentation. Alcohol also reduces the stickiness of blood cells called platelets, and may also increase the ability of blood to dissolve clots. Both these effects may also protect against heart attack.

CASE STUDY: DARREN

Darren, a 39-year-old librarian, is an example of alcohol-related abnormal risk factors. When he first came to the clinic, his cholesterol was high at 7.6, triglycerides were high at 6.7 and HDL was low at 0.8. He had no family history of heart attack or stroke, and had stopped smoking one month before his blood test. He did not exercise regularly. His blood pressure was 160/100 (well above the upper limit of 140/80 for his age). He weighed 82kg with ideal body weight 74kg. He admitted to drinking about 10 litres of sweet white wine a week (an average daily alcohol intake of 14 standard drinks). This was his usual intake for the last five years, but he had noticed no side effects and had never been drunk.

Darren was told he was at increased risk for heart attack because of his abnormal blood fats, overweight and high blood pressure. He was advised to cut back his alcohol to no more than two glasses a day, and walk regularly for at least 20 minutes a day. He was also sent to see a specialist dietitian, who showed that as well as his high alcohol intake Darren had a very high fat intake of 50 per cent of total calories. Darren ate mainly pies, pasties, hot dogs and fish and chips with several slices of bread and butter daily. He was advised to:

- Reduce alcohol
- Reduce fat by almost half
- Reduce sugar
- Eat more wholegrain products (brown rice, pasta, wholemeal bread and cereals), fruit and vegetables

Six weeks later, his weight had fallen to 79kg, and cholesterol was 5.2, triglycerides 1.3 and HDL 0.9. Darren deserved, and received, congratulations.

Three months later, he came back for another check-up. His weight had risen to 82kg; he had increased his wine to five glasses per day, and had stopped walking regularly. His cholesterol level had gone up to 6.7, triglycerides to 2.8 and HDL was 1.0. Darren was referred to a special clinic for further help in controlling his drinking.

Darren's case illustrates the complex relationships between diet, alcohol intake, body weight, levels of blood fats and physical activity. Most of us can change our lifestyle and improve our risk of heart attack.

A glass a day

Current recommendations are for adults to drink on average no more than four standard drinks a day for men and two standard drinks a day for women. But I would suggest about half this amount should provide the benefits with less of the risks. About 75 per cent of adults drink alcohol and most do so without problems. But each year, 20 per cent of the adult population is involved in alcohol-related mental or physical illness, as well as 50 per cent of fatal road accidents.

Many of my colleagues advise their patients to drink a glass of red wine a day to protect against heart disease and to raise HDL levels. There is probably similar benefit from other kinds of alcohol, but an average of 1–2 standard drinks a day is enough.

I see many patients with alcohol-related high triglycerides, central abdominal obesity, low HDL, high blood pressure and diabetes, in whom alcohol restriction is a key part of management. Alcohol intake needs to be monitored and controlled like other factors that can influence risk of heart attack and stroke.

SUMMARY

- Drinking alcohol is a double-edged sword. On the one hand, there are definite health benefits from low alcohol consumption. On the other hand, heavy alcohol consumption is associated with definite health hazards.
- Several mechanisms are responsible for the beneficial effects of alcohol, including raising HDL and anti-oxidant effects.
- There is little evidence that red wine has any greater cardio-protective effect than other forms of alcohol, in spite of red wine containing more anti-oxidants than white.
- 'In moderation' may mean one glass of wine daily to one person, and several glasses daily to another: an average of one standard drink daily for women and two for men is recommended.
- AFDs (alcohol-free days) should be part of your usual routine—at least twice a week.
- Don't drink heavily only on weekends and think you're doing OK because your average for the week is within the guidelines (binge drinking is harmful).
- If you drive, don't drink.
- Alcohol is high in calories and needs to be carefully monitored in a weight-reduction program. On the other hand, one glass of wine may help you stick to your diet, and be a small reward for your self-control.
- Perhaps the advice given over 30 years ago by an old and wise general practitioner of Scottish ancestry is appropriate: 'A whisky a day keeps the heart attacks at bay'. The contemporary advice of a medical colleague may also be appropriate: 'Drink one or two glasses of wine with your evening meal when you feel like it. But don't drink more. Learn to savour your wine, and you will be repaid by better health and a longer life'.

18
For the Love
of Coffee

Now we get to my personal 'pleasure vice'—coffee! My day usually starts with a very weak cup of tea (no more than lightly tinted hot water), which rehydrates me after a good night's sleep. Later, with breakfast, I usually have a cup of skinny *caffe latte,* with super-skim milk (0.1 per cent or virtually no fat content).

Like many millions around the world, I find the coffee gets me off to a good start and focuses my mind on the job ahead. One fine cup of coffee a day is usually all I need. Only rarely do I have a second coffee at around mid-afternoon, when I have a busy evening ahead, perhaps to give a talk or to chair a meeting. Even then, I usually only have a macchiato and just drink half, which is enough to keep me going for the evening, but not enough to keep me awake that night.

I like quality coffee, well made with a nutty flavour, neither bitter nor sour. But like all good things, it's best in moderation, because whether we like to admit it or not, caffeine is a drug. Caffeine is also found in tea, cola drinks and chocolate.

Caffeine and coffee

Caffeine is a member of the *xanthine* family of chemicals, and is one of several ingredients in coffee that has recognised biological actions. Caffeine is a powerful stimulant, increasing both mental alertness and concentration. Within minutes, and lasting for a few hours, there are effects on the heart and blood vessels:

- Increased heart rate
- Increased blood pressure
- Increased blood flow to tissues

Coffee and heart attack

Several early studies showed an association between coffee drinking and increased risk of heart attack:

- In a Boston study in the 1970s, people who drank six or more cups of coffee per day had more than twice the risk of heart attack than those who did not drink coffee.
- In Norway in the 1980s, coronary heart disease risk in male coffee drinkers was twice as high as in non-drinkers.
- The Framingham study reported a higher-than-expected death rate from coronary heart disease in those drinking more than four cups of coffee per day.
- The Physicians Heart Study in the US reported those who drank coffee heavily showed a 2.5-fold higher rate of heart attack than non-drinkers. This association was independent of smoking, age, blood pressure and blood cholesterol levels. Because coffee contains over 300 substances, it was not suggested that caffeine was responsible for the increased risk in coffee drinkers. A limit of two cups of coffee per day was recommended for the average person.

Since these early studies, over 13 further studies compared coffee drinking in people with and without heart attacks. These showed an association between coffee and increased heart attack risk for those drinking three or more cups a day. Ten other studies of people without heart disease at the beginning who were followed up for several years did not show any relationship between developing heart attack and coffee drinking.

Recently it has been shown that the way in which the body metabolises coffee is under genetic control through variation in activity of a liver enzyme called *cytochrome P450 1A*. People with low P450 activity are slow coffee metabolisers and maintain high caffeine blood levels after drinking coffee. They have been shown to be at increased risk of heart attack compared with fast coffee metabolisers who have high P450 activity. Coffee drinking may increase risk of heart attack by raising blood pressure, altering the heart rhythm and blood fats.

Coffee and blood pressure

Blood pressure increases in proportion to the number of cups of coffee per day. A single cup of coffee may acutely increase systolic blood pressure by up to 10 mmHg.

Coffee and palpitations

Many people experience palpitations following coffee or tea; these are caused by caffeine intake stimulating the heart. Excessive coffee drinking may also increase the risk of death from an abnormal heart rhythm, possibly because caffeine releases adrenaline and noradrenaline.

Coffee and blood fats

Several studies have shown the relationship between coffee and increased cholesterol, triglyceride and LDL levels. Several other studies, however, have not shown an association between coffee consumption and blood cholesterol levels.

The way coffee is prepared affects its cholesterol-raising properties. Boiling coffee, a practice common in Scandinavia, extracts a greater amount of the substances responsible for raising LDL. These are called *cafestol* and *kahweol*, and belong to the family of substances called *diterpenes*. Steaming coffee (as in Italian coffee machines) extracts less of these diterpenes and has less effect on LDL. In addition, cafestol occurs in both Robusta and Arabica varieties of coffee beans, while kahweol occurs only in Arabica. Kahweol is less potent than cafestol in raising LDL, so that Arabica coffee has also less LDL-raising potential than Robusta coffee. Filtering coffee through paper removes much of the cafestol and kahweol and has little effect on LDL levels.

Recommendations for drinking coffee

1. Limit your coffees to a maximum of two cups per day, especially if you have high blood pressure, abnormal blood fats, abnormal heart rhythm, and have suffered previous heart attack or stroke.

2. We don't know yet the effects on heart attack and stroke of coffee substitutes made from non-caffeine-containing vegetable products, such as rye, barley, chicory, broad beans, malted barley and sugar beet. Therefore, we can't make recommendations.

3. Caffeine also occurs in relatively large amounts in tea, chocolate and cola-containing soft drinks, so if you have a history of coronary disease, it is best to limit your intake of these foods.

SUMMARY

- Coffee contains substances with recognised effects on the heart and blood vessels and blood fats.
- The results linking coffee drinking to increased heart attacks are inconclusive, but recent genetic studies suggest that if you metabolise caffeine slowly, you may be at increased risk.
- Have your coffee and enjoy it—once or twice a day!

19
Controlling Those Carbs

'Carbs' is a relatively new buzz-word in our society. We are becoming more and more 'carb-conscious', aware of the so-called good or complex carbohydrates and somewhat cautious about the simple or 'empty' carbs. We read about the special diets of elite athletes and we think about enhancing our normal energy performance by choosing what we believe will help us get through our busy days.

This is not a bad thing, as the more we know about foods with which to fuel our bodies, the better choices we're likely to make.

What are carbs?

The word *carbohydrate* refers to substances with the chemical composition (carbon + hydrogen + oxygen). These are the ingredients the body uses to make carbohydrates, which provide energy for its metabolic processes. Glucose and glycogen are the body's major carbohydrates.

Simple carbs (sugars)

These include glucose, sucrose (cane sugar), fructose (fruit sugar) and maltose. High-sugar intakes are typical of the diet of Western industrial countries, as are the intakes of high saturated fat and cholesterol. Sugars are called *simple carbs* because they have a relatively simple chemical structure, are easily digested and absorbed, and are readily converted by the body into glucose (the sugar used by the body for energy).

Complex carbs

Complex carbs, on the other hand, have a complex chemical structure. They include plant fibres and glycogen, which comprises a long chain of glucose molecules.

Glycogen acts as the body's energy storage of carbs, particularly in muscle fibres, which use glucose to supply energy for contraction and therefore movement of the body.

Plant fibres are more slowly digested and absorbed than the simple carbs. They provide bulk in the diet through their high-fibre content, and are necessary for normal bowel function.

Carbohydrate balance: simple vs. complex

Carbohydrates provide about 40 per cent of energy requirements for most people, although this is close to 45 per cent in teenagers and 35 per cent in older adults. Soft drinks supply about 25 per cent of energy requirements in teenagers compared with 10 per cent in older adults, who eat more fruit. Other sources of sugars include cakes, buns, jams, honey, sweet desserts, sweet biscuits, confectionery, chocolate and added sugar.

Complex carbs (mostly cereals and vegetables) supply about 15–20 per cent of total energy.

What is dietary fibre?

Dietary fibre is of plant origin and refers to non-digestible carbs and related substances. There are three main types of dietary fibre:

- Cellulose (a complex carb made up of glucose sub-units)
- Lignin (part of the woody stem of plants)
- Others (pectins, gums, mucilages and hemicellulose)

The 'others' are important sources of energy because they are fermented in the intestine by bacteria, producing gas and short-chain-length fatty acids. These fatty acids are capable of providing a significant proportion of dietary energy.

Does dietary fibre affect blood cholesterol?

Several studies have shown that blood cholesterol levels are reduced in response to a high-fibre intake, although the effectiveness of each type of fibre varies. Lignin, gums, mucilages and hemicellulose also bind to bile salts in the intestine and reduce their absorption. This may result in a slight lowering of blood cholesterol levels.

Populations with a high-fibre intake have low rates of coronary heart disease. These groups also tend to eat few simple carbs, and have a low intake of cholesterol and saturated fats.

What about other blood fats?

A high intake of sugars can raise blood cholesterol and triglyceride levels and reduce HDL. This commonly leads to overweight and diabetes, and the risk of heart attack is also increased.

In some people, triglycerides are very sensitive to the amount of sugar in the diet. Even a normal intake of sugars can result in high triglycerides in carb-sensitive individuals.

Low HDL and high cholesterol are often associated with these high blood triglyceride levels and significantly increase the risk of heart attack.

Alcohol and blood fats

Alcohol consumption (especially in carb-sensitive people) may also raise levels of cholesterol and triglycerides.

Dietary recommendations

In the US, the recommended intake of energy from all forms of carbs is 55–60 per cent, with sugars providing about 15 per cent and complex carbs 50–45 per cent. This compares with the normal Australian diet in which carbs supply about 44 per cent of total energy, sugars 27 per cent and complex carbs a very low 17 per cent. The low complex carb intake in the Australian diet is reflected in an average fibre intake of 10–15g per day (the recommended minimal daily amount is 15–20g).

Current recommendations are to reduce sugars and increase fibre intake:

- Reduce consumption of sugar-containing, low-fibre foods such as cakes, buns, sweets and biscuits.
- Don't add sugar to tea, coffee or cereals.
- Don't use sweetened fruit juices.
- Eat wholemeal cereals and bread.
- Increase intake of fruit and vegetables.

These simple measures will re-educate your palate to get used to unsweetened foods. Look out for sweetened foods by reading the labels.

Many products, particularly breakfast cereals and 'low-fat' foods, have high sugar content. Read the labels! A typical example of commercial muesli, made predominantly of oats, whole grains, nuts and fruits, contains about 17 per cent by weight of sugars and 13 per cent of fibre. The order of ingredients by weight is oats, dried fruit, wheat bran, wheat germ, raw sugar and honey. You can see why this muesli tastes so sugary! Many low-fat types of yoghurt are also loaded with sugar, especially those with fruit. See Part VII: Low–Chol Cuisine for some tasty recipes for homemade muesli and other low-sugar, cholesterol-lowering foods.

Carbs are also involved in diabetes and the metabolic syndrome (see Chapter 21). These are conditions in which blood glucose levels tend to be high.

SUMMARY

- The body uses sugars as a readily available source of energy.
- The body uses complex carbs in the form of glycogen to store energy.
- Plant fibres in the diet can also be an important source of energy by being converted by bacteria in the intestine to fatty acids.
- Plant fibres are important for normal bowel function.
- Most people's diet is woefully low on fibre intake and greatly exceeds the recommended intake of sugars.
- Eat low-sugar and high-fibre foods to help control blood fats and reduce risk of heart attack and stroke.

20
Flab is Not Fab

Losing weight is one of the most commonly discussed topics in our society. Visit your nearest bookshop and you'll notice that one of the biggest sections in the lifestyle section is devoted to diet and weight loss.

They say one-third of the population is on a diet, one-third is about to go on a diet—and one-third ought to be on a diet!

Certainly, the health profession is currently very concerned about the overweight epidemic and the illnesses that accompany it. Excessive weight is now the big health challenge for government and for the health industry.

Over many years, population studies have shown that weight gain is a major factor contributing to heart attack and stroke. Weight gain may be associated with several risk factors:

- Cholesterol increases
- LDL and triglycerides increase
- HDL falls
- Blood pressure increases

Other changes affect the body in different ways:

- The heart beats faster, even when at rest.
- Overweight people are less able to exercise, and when they do, their heart beats faster.

- Their bodies need higher levels of insulin to maintain blood glucose levels, and diabetes is more common (see Chapter 21).

All of these changes show the body's normal functions are impaired by weight gain.

Weight gain is usually slow, insidious and unnoticed until we need to let out our belts, buy larger sizes, or until someone remarks on our larger clothing size. This is not usually taken as a compliment!

Because fat is stored inside the body as well as under the skin, looking at overall body weight tends to underestimate the amount of fat tissue that the body has produced.

For example, a 70kg man has a fat tissue mass of about 10.5kg. Water, bone and muscle account for most of the rest. If this man increases his weight by 10 per cent to 77kg by increasing his body fat tissue to 17.5kg, the increase in his fat tissue mass has been 70 per cent. The body's fat metabolism is disturbed considerably.

Weight gain leads to higher levels of blood cholesterol and triglycerides and lower HDL levels. Looking at the relationship between overweight and heart attacks, therefore, we would expect to find that heart attacks are more frequent in those who are overweight.

This is indeed the case, as shown in several studies. For example, in the Framingham study:
- Angina occurred 2–3 times more frequently in those who were 20 per cent above average weight compared to those whose weight was 10 per cent below average.
- Sudden death was four times more frequent in the 20 per cent overweight group.
- For each 10 per cent gain in weight in men and women there was an increase of about 6.5 in systolic blood pressure and 0.33 in blood cholesterol levels.

Life insurance statistics have also shown a strong relationship between excessive death rates and degree of overweight.

- The average death rate is associated with normal body mass indices (BMI) between 20 and 25, with BMI being calculated by weight (kg) divided by the square of height (metres).
- Death rates increase by 50 per cent at a BMI of 32.
- Death rates increase by 100 per cent at a BMI of 36.
- Death rates increase by 150 per cent at a BMI of 38.

You can check your own BMI by referring to the weight for height chart in Figure 20.1. The healthy weight range applies to BMI between 20 and 25. Overweight refers to BMI between 25 and 30; people above 30 BMI are obese. Underweight people have BMI below 20.

Figure 20.1. Weight for height chart.

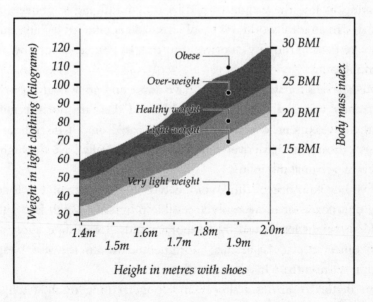

Such is the extent of weight gain in our community that it is now regarded as an epidemic that is likely to result in a massive health burden in the years ahead—from diabetes, arthritis and cardiovascular disease.

The good news

Many of the effects of overweight are reversible:

- For every 10 per cent loss in weight, there are similar falls in systolic blood pressure and blood cholesterol levels.
- People previously diagnosed with diabetes can restore blood glucose levels to normal after weight loss.
- Weight loss can also raise protective HDL levels.

Losing weight

A billion-dollar weight-loss industry has become established to fight flab in Western countries. Diet books on weight loss abound and are almost always found at the top of bestseller lists.

Tragically, while millions are starving, other millions are paying huge amounts to lose the weight gained by over-indulging in unnecessary calories. In an ideal world this would instead be spent on feeding those who are getting too few calories—but that, of course, is not how it is working out.

Medications for weight control have come and gone over the years. Currently very few drugs are available, and they are not subsidised by the government. Weight loss is mostly based on self-discipline. Of course, those who have over-indulged do not usually have the highest levels of personal discipline.

If you or your doctor think you need to lose weight you can follow one of a dozen or more easily accessible programs. We all know that sudden weight loss is usually temporary, and after a huge effort and sometimes spectacular results, most people regain the lost weight within six months. I have seen it time and again.

Far better to aim at a slower and longer-lasting result. I tell my patients weight loss is easy. Simply eat less and exercise more. How easy is that? Well, in truth it is not easy at all. Food is one of our most basic rewards. We work hard and then we reward ourselves with a drink or two and a huge meal, followed by a nice long sleep. Sounds reasonable, but it is a recipe for stacking on the kilos. They used to say that to stay trim, one needed to breakfast like a king, lunch like a prince and dine like a pauper. That's OK for those with time to digest a huge breakfast, time to sit down to a substantial lunch followed by a nap and then be too full in the evening to even consider more than a light snack. But it does not fit in with the normal working day.

Most of us have our main meal of the day in the evening. We should therefore be aware of what we have for the meal and make it rewarding in colour, taste and texture, but not high in kilojoules. There are dozens of recipe books that will help you re-think your meals. Pick those that suit your taste and lifestyle.

In general terms, the simplest way to lose weight is to cut back the calories, particularly those empty calories that have no nutritional value, such as fizzy sugary drinks, cakes, biscuits and pastries.

Anyone seriously contemplating weight loss of more than a few kilos should see a competent dietitian who will work out a tailor-made eating program and often suggest a suitable exercise program to go along with it, or refer you on to a trained exercise instructor. The calculation is simple: put less in, work off more and you will end up slimmer and trimmer (and indeed fitter).

A dietitian consultation can help you work towards a target weight and then maintain it.

A few hints, however, will help if you are just planning to shed a few extra kilos if you are slightly over your ideal body weight.

- Drink plenty of water. You'll be surprised at how often, when you reach for the bread and cheese, what you are actually experiencing is thirst not hunger. You should drink a glass of cool but not cold water—slowly. Wait ten minutes. If you are still hungry then eat, but not before.
- Cut out extra fat, e.g. never put 'spread' of any kind on your bread or toast, use fat-free milk and dairy products.
- Refrain from putting sugar in hot drinks such as tea and coffee.
- Never eat between meals. So simple, but very effective. Eat three suitably low-calorie meals a day and have snacks

mid-morning and mid-afternoon.

- Never, ever eat after 8pm. Not even a single peanut. If you adopt this one strategy you will be surprised how much weight you lose and keep off.
- If you adopt a low-chol eating plan you will almost certainly lose weight, even without trying.
- Eat slowly. We all eat much too fast and food is made easy to eat. If we had to work harder at getting at our food we'd eat more slowly and know earlier if we were full. Often we only 'feel' full long after we *are* full, because it takes a while for us to experience the full feeling. By eating slowly you will be more aware of your satiation point. Eat as if you were at a dinner party, even if you are alone. Fast eaters tend to be overweight, so just by slowing down your eating you will be likely to lose some weight.

SUMMARY

- Weight gain has reached epidemic proportions in Australia, the UK and the US. Overweight is almost the norm.
- Weight gain in children leads to overweight adults— establish healthy eating habits and exercise early.
- Fats, sugars and alcohol are high-energy culprits that should be limited for weight control.
- Weight loss improves a range of risk factors from blood pressure and insulin levels to HDL and LDL.
- Weight loss can prevent and control adult-onset diabetes.

21
Blood Glucose Disorders

It is important to take note of disorders that cause high blood sugar. Not only do they cause clogging of the arteries, they also damage the small blood vessels of the eye and kidneys. The most serious of these are diabetes and the metabolic syndrome.

Diabetes and the metabolic syndrome are conditions in which the body's metabolism of glucose and insulin are abnormal. The two conditions overlap, and a person can move from one to the other and back again depending on body weight and other factors.

Weight gain is increasing in epidemic proportions in Western societies, some Asian countries and indeed most places where people are well fed.

The same is true of diabetes and the metabolic syndrome, which are both related to weight gain, and are both effectively controlled using modern medication.

Diabetes

The full name for diabetes is *diabetes mellitus*. People with diabetes tend to have high blood sugar (glucose) levels and they need to avoid sugars and sweets.

There are two kinds of diabetes: insulin-dependent or juvenile diabetes (Type 1 diabetes) and non-insulin-dependent or mature-onset diabetes (Type 2 diabetes).

Type 1 diabetes
People with Type 1 diabetes have low levels of insulin because the beta cells in the pancreas, which produce insulin, are malfunctioning. These people require regular insulin and are usually children or young adults with a genetic predisposition.

Type 2 diabetes
Other diabetics do not need insulin injections and in fact have higher insulin levels than normal. They are able to control their blood glucose levels by diet or tablets, are usually adults, and are called either mature-onset, non insulin-dependent or Type 2 diabetics. Type 2 is far more common than Type 1, and is more related to being overweight.

The diabetes epidemic
Because weight gain is a problem in most Western as well as many developing and Eastern populations, diabetes is becoming alarmingly common all over the world—so much so that diabetes is now a disease of epidemic proportions.

The metabolic syndrome
A syndrome is a group of clinical abnormalities that commonly occur together. The metabolic syndrome has also been called the *central obesity syndrome*, the *insulin-resistance syndrome*, and *Reaven's syndrome* after the physician who first described its features.

The basic underlying feature of the metabolic syndrome is the release of excessive amounts of insulin by the pancreas in an attempt to keep blood glucose levels in the normal range.

The metabolic syndrome may be regarded as a pre-diabetic condition, and a person may progress over several years to diabetes, as their body's metabolism of glucose and insulin becomes increasingly abnormal, often in association with progressive weight gain.

The metabolic syndrome is related to weight gain as a result of fat accumulating within the abdomen—so-called *central abdominal fat* or *visceral fat* surrounding the internal organs. There are several definitions of the metabolic syndrome.

The US definition requires at least three of the following:

- Waist circumference greater than 102cm in men and 88cm in women.
- Fasting triglycerides of 1.7 or more.
- Fasting HDL less than 1.04 in men and 1.29 in women.
- Blood pressure greater than 130/85.
- Fasting blood glucose 6 or more.

In the US, the metabolic syndrome increases with age from about 5–10 per cent of those aged 20–30 to 40–45 per cent of those aged over 60. Overall it occurs in about one in four people.

Weight gain and the metabolic syndrome

Diabetes and the metabolic syndrome are conditions in which the body's metabolism of glucose and insulin are abnormal.

There is some degree of overlap between these conditions because, depending on diet and exercise levels, a person may belong to any one class for a certain period of time but shift to another for another period.

It is possible to swing back to the same disorder more than once over several years. For example, a person's glucose metabolism can return to normal, usually with strict weight control through diet and exercise, in spite of previously being diabetic. Furthermore, progression diabetes may be prevented by avoiding weight gain.

There is a clear and consistent relationship between weight gain and abnormal glucose metabolism, which may well explain the epidemic of diabetes in our community.

How common are disorders of glucose metabolism?

Disorders of glucose metabolism are occurring much more frequently in Western and other populations, especially indigenous populations including New Zealand Maoris, Australian Aborigines and Torres Strait Islanders. The increase is in epidemic proportions as these populations gain weight.

Increased cardiovascular risk in carbohydrate disorders

Diabetes and the metabolic syndrome increase the risk of heart attack, stroke and other vascular disease for several reasons:

- Blood levels of LDL and triglycerides are often high and HDL low.
- High glucose and insulin levels lead to thickening of the arteries, partly through accumulation of collagen and elastin.
- There is increased trapping in the artery wall of LDL and other damaging substances.

All these changes play a role in clogging of the arteries. The rate of fatal heart attack in Type 2 diabetics is 2–5 times higher than in non-diabetics of the same age, and is similar to people who have already had a heart attack. For this reason, Type 2 diabetes is called a *coronary risk equivalent* disorder.

The metabolic syndrome is also associated with greater risk of heart attack. A study in Finland showed that 51-year-old men with the metabolic syndrome had a three times higher rate of death from heart attack and a doubled risk of death from all causes than men who did not have the metabolic syndrome.

What causes metabolic syndrome and diabetes?

Many factors interact to cause these conditions. Essentially, they are caused by an imbalance of the body's handling of carbohydrates through impaired insulin activity and excessive storage of fat in the fat

144

tissues, liver and muscle.

The factors responsible for these metabolic problems include lack of physical exercise, excessive consumption of simple carbohydrates, hormone imbalance, and genetic factors.

Excessive visceral (abdominal) fat is a hallmark of these conditions. Visceral fat is quite different from fat elsewhere in the body such as the fat layer under the skin (subcutaneous fat) because visceral fat is more metabolically active, is deposited more rapidly and can be lost more quickly. For example, a 5–10 per cent loss of body weight can result in up to 30 per cent loss of visceral fat stores because the body sheds visceral fat in preference to subcutaneous fat.

Visceral fat occurs amongst people who are inactive; who have a diet high in cordials, soft drinks, sugars and fats; and who don't eat enough fibre, fruit and vegetables.

Visceral fat converts hormones made by the adrenal gland into cortisol, and also delivers excessive amounts of fatty acids to the liver, which converts them to triglycerides. Some of these are released into the blood, thereby raising blood triglyceride levels.

Drugs for the metabolic syndrome and diabetes

Several drugs are used to lower blood fats and reduce the risk of diabetes and the metabolic syndrome.

Doctors now regularly prescribe statins for diabetics because these drugs have been shown to lower the risk of heart attack and stroke in both diabetics and non-diabetics. Statins are drugs to lower cholesterol, especially LDL (see Chapter 31).

SUMMARY

- For every recognised diabetic, there is an unrecognised one.
- The number of diabetics has tripled since 1981.
- The proportion of diabetics with abnormal coronary risk factors is higher than in non-diabetics.
- High blood pressure is three times more common in diabetics than in non-diabetics (it occurs in 69 per cent).
- High triglycerides are three times more common (it occurs in 44 per cent).
- Low HDL is twice as common (it occurs in 23 per cent).
- Diabetes shortens life expectancy by up to 15 years through cardiovascular disease and kidney failure.
- Diabetes is a major cause of blindness.
- The rate of fatal heart attack is 2–5 times higher in diabetics than in non-diabetics of the same age, and is similar to people who have already had a heart attack. For this reason, Type 2 diabetes is called a *coronary risk equivalent* disorder.
- Risk factor control is a high priority for Type 2 diabetics: this means no smoking, lose weight, keep LDL and blood pressure low and consider treatment with aspirin. Aspirin is an anti-inflammatory drug that also thins the blood by reducing the activity of platelets in the blood. Aspirin reduces the risk of heart attacks and strokes in those with previous vascular disorders, and diabetics are now more commonly taking it.
- Treatment with statins is necessary for diabetics, regardless of blood fat levels, in view of lower heart attack and stroke rates shown in clinical trials with statins.
- Diabetics should also be considered for treatment with fenofibrate in view of benefits shown for damage to the eyes and kidneys. Statins can be taken safely with fenofibrate by most people.

22
Prohibited and Forbidden: Cigarettes

Let me be crystal clear on this issue. I, like most modern health professionals, do not have a single good word to say about cigarette smoking. Most doctors consider it to be the most destructive legal drug available in our society. Cigarette smoking remains the most important preventable cause of death and disability in Western societies. Let's repeat that: *the single most important preventable cause of death and disability.*

When cigarette smoking became universally popular in the early part of last century, the long-term side effects were not known. Its short-term, acute side effects were disregarded—smelly breath and hair, discoloured teeth and skin, loss of taste and smell, eye and respiratory tract irritation, and nausea and palpitations in those starting to smoke.

In the last 60 or so years, the links between cigarette smoking and the development of heart attack, stroke, chronic lung disease and lung cancer have become progressively stronger. There is now no doubt that cigarette smoking is a causative factor in these diseases, and there is no doubt that lung diseases can be largely prevented by avoiding cigarette smoke.

Death rates from heart attack and sudden death are directly related to the number of cigarettes smoked for both men and women. Heavy smokers have five times the death rate from heart attack than non-smokers.

Passive smoking

Passive smoking refers to inhaling others' smoke. It can lead to:

- Acute asthma in susceptible people.
- Angina (chest pain due to lack of blood supply to the heart muscle) in people with clogging of the coronary arteries.
- Increased risk of heart attack.
- Higher rates of bronchitis and pneumonia in children of smoking parents.

Side-stream smoke coming from a burning cigarette sitting on a table or in an ash-tray has:

- Five times more carbon monoxide than mainstream smoke inhaled directly into a smoker's lungs.
- Twice more tar and nicotine than mainstream smoke. This means a non-smoker sitting in a smoke-filled room for eight hours inhales the equivalent of two cigarettes.

The older adult population is still giving up smoking and being immediately rewarded by improvement in the sense of taste and smell, improvement in respiratory and cardiovascular function, and saving of immediate costs.

Smoking and heart attacks

How does smoking increase the risk of heart attacks and sudden death? Several mechanisms have been suggested:

- The blood tends to clot more easily.
- Nicotine also increases the excitability of heart muscle and increases the risk of ventricular fibrillation, an abnormal heart rhythm that causes sudden death.
- HDL is lowered sufficiently to account for a significant component of the increased risk.

Why do people continue to smoke?

Many say it's relaxing. Others say it's because they put on weight when they try to stop. But in a study of over 100 men and women, the average weight gain over three months in those stopping smoking was only 1.5kg. Paying attention to diet and increasing physical activity will help you control weight gain.

Unlike all other age groups where fewer people are smoking, increasing numbers of young women are taking up smoking. Peer pressure and the desire to look mature and sophisticated may be the main reasons. If only these young women knew how silly they looked! Nicotine dependence is a major reason for people continuing to smoke.

Quitting

'Giving up smoking is the easiest thing in the world. I know because I've given it up thousands of times.' —Mark Twain

What the author of *Tom Sawyer* didn't say was that stopping smoking lowers the risk of heart attack significantly within one or two years, partly due to a rise in HDL levels, decreases the clotting tendency of the blood, and other effects.

Nicotine dependence

Cigarette smokers are 'hooked' on nicotine—it's a drug of dependence (in other words, physical withdrawal symptoms and signs occur when it is withdrawn, and there is also a psychological dependence on the drug).

How dependent on nicotine are you?

Question	Answer	Points
How soon after you wake do you have your first cigarette?	Within 5 min 6–30 min 30–60 min after 60 min	3 2 1 0
Is it difficult to refrain from smoking in places where it is banned?	Yes No	1 0
Which cigarette would you most hate to give up?	The first one in the morning Any other	1 0
How many cigarettes a day do you smoke?	31 or more 21–30 11–20 10 or less	3 2 1 0
Do you smoke more in the first few hours of the day than during the rest of the day?	Yes No	1 0
Do you smoke if you are ill in bed?	Yes No	1 0

Nicotine dependence: your results
High: 6–10 points
Medium–high: 4–7 points
Low–medium: 1–5 points

Withdrawal symptoms

People who stop smoking often complain of headache, irritability, difficulty in sleeping and increased tension. These symptoms are largely due to nicotine withdrawal. Nicotine is addictive and has powerful actions on the heart, nervous system and many other body tissues:

- Nicotine increases blood pressure and heart rate, stimulates heart muscle to contract more strongly, and increases the tendency for the heart muscle to develop abnormalities in rhythm.
- Nicotine increases platelet stickiness and the blood-clotting tendency, and increases the release of the hormones adrenaline and noradrenaline into the

bloodstream. These hormones cause the increased heart rate with cigarette smoking.

You can prevent some nicotine withdrawal symptoms by using either nicotine-containing chewing gum, or by nicotine skin patches. But if you have high blood pressure, stomach ulcers, overactive thyroid, diabetes and kidney failure, nicotine must be used cautiously as it may aggravate these conditions.

Zyban
Zyban is a recently available drug that helps overcome nicotine dependence. Do not use nicotine patches and gums if you are on Zyban. Zyban is not suitable for people with certain neurological disorders or who are taking certain drugs—check with your doctor.

What else should I do when quitting?
Some people tend to put on weight. While watching the calories is important, a change to the low-fat, low-sugar, low-cholesterol and high complex carbohydrate diet will help (see Part VII: Low-Chol Cuisine). You should also increase your exercise.

SUMMARY

- Young people with clogging of the arteries are almost invariably smokers.
- Diabetic smokers are particularly prone to clogging of the arteries in the legs. Amputation is virtually confined to smokers.
- When quitting, you might need help overcoming your nicotine addiction such as patches or a quit program.
- Rapid benefits follow from quitting—within months, cardiovascular risk drops by almost 50 per cent.
- After quitting, tastebuds recover and food tastes good again.

23

The Fitness Factor

Let's look at the Big E: Exercise. Exercise is one of the best things we can do for ourselves. Not only will we help our bones, our muscles, and our cardiovascular system, but also those who exercise regularly feel better and look better.

If I could prescribe a magic pill which would make you lose weight, reshape your body, improve the colour of your skin, lift your mood and even create social experiences for you, you'd race out and buy a huge container of my pills. Well, the magic pill you need—and it really is magic—is regular, enjoyable exercise.

You were issued a healthy body at birth. Use it or lose it, it is as simple as that. You only have to look at children in a playground. They are like puppies running around all over the place—just for the pleasure of the movement, for the fun of using their bodies.

In adulthood, unless we are careful, we can lose this pleasurable form of activity. Our bodies suffer, and so we exercise even less. This creates a vicious cycle of unhealthy non-activity. Don't let it happen to you!

You won't wear out by doing moderate exercise. There's no truth in the rumour that our hearts are only capable of a certain number of heartbeats. Our heart, lungs and muscles are designed for exercise. Not that this is evident from population surveys.

Couch potatoes

About one in six adults are sedentary—they don't have any form of physical activity. Only half are undertaking enough exercise to maintain good health.

Lack of exercise is a definite risk factor for heart and vascular diseases. For example, in the Framingham study, fit men had half the death rate from these diseases as unfit men (see Table 23.1).

Table 23.1. Cardiovascular death rates according to age and exercise levels.

Exercise level	Age 35–44 y	Age 45–54y	Age 55–64y
Very low	3.5	12.6	22.5
Low	4	10.5	19.1
Medium	1.8	10.2	12
High	1.4	9.6	9.1

Benefits of exercise

One of the first studies to show a benefit from exercise was the famous bus conductors' study in London. Heart attack rates were lower in bus conductors compared with drivers, and the difference was attributed to variation in exercise levels.

A lower rate of heart attack, sudden death and angina has been found in many other studies. Again, let's look at the Framingham study:

- Sudden death was almost four times lower in fitter men.
- Angina was about 50 per cent lower in fitter men.

One reason for the benefits of exercise on heart health is a change in blood fat levels:

- Blood triglycerides, cholesterol and LDL are lower in physically conditioned people.
- HDL levels are also higher, especially in extremely fit people like marathon runners.

CASE STUDY: LYN

Lyn is a non-smoking, non-drinking, 40-year-old woman who works at a gym. She runs an average of 10km a day and is 4kg below her ideal body weight. Her first blood test showed high cholesterol at 6.5. Other blood fats were: HDL 3.5, triglycerides 0.3 and LDL 3.0. In spite of her high cholesterol, Lyn has a low risk of heart attack because of her extremely high HDL levels.

There are at least three reasons for Lyn's high blood HDL level.

1. Women have higher HDL levels than men (mainly because HDL levels in men are reduced by the male hormone, testosterone).

2. She has a high level of physical fitness, which is associated with high HDL levels.

3. Lyn's parents both lived into their nineties. Lyn may have a genetically high blood HDL level, which may be increased further by her level of physical fitness.

Lyn is an example of exercise-related, hormone-related, and possibly genetically determined high HDL.

CASE STUDY: JOHN

John enrolled in a get-fit exercise program, with twice-weekly periods of jogging for 20 minutes, preceded by a 10-minute warm-up period and followed by another 10-minute cool-down period. No advice was given on weight, diet or smoking habits.

After 12 weeks John lost 10.6kg in weight, reduced his skin fat thickness by about 50 per cent, improved his exercise capacity by 25 per cent, reduced alcohol consumption from ten glasses of beer to four glasses daily, and cut smoking by half.

His cholesterol fell by 35 per cent, his LDL by 30 per cent, and his triglycerides by 58 per cent. John's HDL increased by 7 per cent. His exercise program and changing alcohol and smoking habits were responsible for the improvement in his blood fats.

John's response is typical of people going on a prolonged exercise program. Not only does their body metabolism change with exercise but also their other lifestyle habits often change as well.

The body's response to exercise

Regular exercise improves the body's capacity to cope with emotional as well as physical stress. People who take up a fitness program tend to find that they don't need alcohol and tobacco to relax as much as they did before they started exercising.

Some people also experience a change in personality as they become fitter. Regular exercisers appear to have a more positive attitude to life than those who don't exercise. Studies of regular joggers have shown that they are more self-sufficient, forthright and imaginative; are less depressed, less hypochondriacal (less concerned about their own body's symptoms); have a better self-image and are more efficient workers than non-joggers.

Regular exercisers have been shown to be able to concentrate for longer periods, have a faster mental response, more originality of thought, increased mental tenacity, the ability to carry more than one idea at the same time, and are able to change from one subject to another more quickly than those who do not exercise regularly. The physically fit body responds differently to many sorts of stimuli than the non-physically fit.

One important alteration with fitness is the response to stressful stimuli. We are all familiar with the rapid heartbeat associated with fright, fear, or acute emotional upset, or after running fast for a short distance. This increased heart rate is a normal response of the sympathetic nervous system to stimulation—the classic 'fright or flight' response described years ago by the famous Canadian physiologist Hans Selye. While this response is designed to be a protective one, readying the body for defence or aggression, it also may be harmful and indeed fatal. Being 'frightened to death' is a well-recognised phenomenon, and many anecdotes have described people dropping dead after a sudden shock or fright.

Recent studies have shown that physically fit people have a much smaller rise in heart rate than unfit people in response to stimulation of the sympathetic nervous system. This 'attenuated response' in the physically fit may protect their hearts from over-stimulation and from sudden death.

Another important change in the physically fit involves increased capacity of the body to deal with ingested fat, sugar and cholesterol. All are handled more efficiently, with more rapid return to normal levels after such food is eaten.

Exercise appears to work by increasing the activity of the enzyme *lipoprotein lipase*, which is responsible for breaking down triglycerides in the bloodstream. Lipoprotein lipase occurs on the endothelial lining of capillary vessels in the lungs, liver, heart, skeletal muscle and fatty (adipose) tissue.

Taking care when exercising

Exercise can be dangerous where there is severe underlying coronary heart disease, particularly in the previously inactive person who suddenly takes up unaccustomed exercise.

Sudden death is a rare complication; about 4–5 per cent of cases of sudden death are related to unaccustomed or unduly strenuous physical activity. Most are due to abnormal heart rhythm with underlying severe coronary artery disease, and plaque rupture is the most common underlying cause. Because of the small risk of sudden death with unaccustomed exercise, any exercise program undertaken by people who may have silent coronary heart disease must be supervised and begun very slowly.

An exercise stress test is recommended for inactive people aged 35 years or above before beginning an exercise program, particularly if they have known coronary risk factors such as hypertension, high blood cholesterol levels, or are cigarette smokers.

Tailoring an exercise program

Each exercise program needs to be tailored to an individual's needs. There are several important points to consider:

- Our capacity for physical exercise decreases progressively with age, as does the average maximum heart rate that we can achieve. The maximum heart rate is about 220-age (beats per minute).
- Those who have previously been inactive should begin exercising at no more than 70 per cent (ideally 50–60 per cent) of maximum heart rate.
- The exercise should be preceded by a slow warm-up period, including muscle stretching, which will reduce the tendency for ligament and tendon damage.
- Initially, the exercise period should be short (10–15 minutes) and every second or third day.
- Older people are often limited in the amount of exercise they can do because of joint problems caused by wear and tear (osteoarthritis). Pain relievers, physiotherapy and other treatments may be necessary before regular exercise is possible.
- Aerobic exercises are recommended for cardiovascular fitness. These are exercises that require a steady supply of oxygen for continued muscle activity, and include walking, jogging, running, swimming, cycling and cross-country skiing.
- Choose the best type of aerobic exercise for you: the one that you enjoy most and are most likely to continue over a prolonged period, and the most convenient to your lifestyle.

Walking

The older person often chooses walking, which is safe, can be undertaken almost anywhere without special equipment and which allows you to see and enjoy the scenery as you go past.

Jogging

Younger people often choose jogging, which builds up physical fitness very rapidly and also needs minimum equipment. It is very important for joggers to have proper running shoes to prevent ligament and joint injury, and to increase the level of exercise slowly.

Swimming

Swimming is in many ways ideal, for it is more strenuous than jogging and causes relatively few tendon, ligament and joint problems. Ready access to a suitable pool can be a problem, however, particularly in colder climates.

Cycling

Cycling is also a very effective way to increase cardiovascular fitness, irrespective of how sophisticated the actual bicycle is. Proper equipment is important, however, particularly cycling helmets and identification tags, lights, flags and other devices that warn approaching traffic of the cyclist's presence on the road. Many countries are now beginning to provide bicycle tracks alongside main roads, considerably increasing the safety of cycling.

Enjoy!

Exercise should be an enjoyable part of everyday life. Already in the US there are over 30 million regular joggers; almost half the adult population does regular exercise of some sort. The number of regular joggers has increased from about 100,000 in 1968 to the enormous number it is today.

Most people feel better after exercise and cope better with the stresses of daily life.

Long, slow, distance

The key to any successful aerobics program is *long, slow, distance*. With progressive training you can slowly increase your distances of cycling, walking, jogging or swimming. Speed does not matter. It is far better to go at a slow and steady pace without getting exhausted, puffed out or experiencing muscle and joint pains, than to try to speed up. With increasing fitness you will speed up without realising it, because you will be able to exercise at lower heart rates, with less sensation of exhaustion or strain.

Age and exercise

Anyone, regardless of age or sex, can undertake safe aerobic exercise even from a sedentary level. Depending on the condition of the joints and muscles, and the severity of underlying coronary artery disease, even elderly people can achieve high levels of physical fitness.

Resting heart rate

As you become fitter, your resting heart rate (RHR) will decrease. Extremely fit athletes have RHR below 50 beats per minute, and occasionally below 40. This compares with average RHR in adults of about 70–80. Aerobic conditioning will drop RHR by about 15 beats per minute after three months, in men and women.

- Exercise lowers our RHR because the heart muscle increases in size, strength and efficiency, and the volume of blood pumped increases. Therefore, a given volume of blood can be delivered to the resting body at a lower heart rate. Furthermore, exercise lowers the activity of the sympathetic nervous system. This system stimulates the pacemaker of the heart, and increased sympathetic tone (for example, in response to exercise or emotion) results in increased pacemaker activity and increased heart rate.
- Recently, a low RHR has been shown to be a protective risk factor against coronary heart disease. People with low RHR developed coronary heart disease at a lower rate than people with high RHR. The protection of the low RHR was independent of other coronary risk factors (including blood cholesterol and HDL levels, blood pressure, age,

sex, and degree of overweight). The RHR did, as expected, correlate with the level of physical activity.

Improving risk factors with exercise

The following coronary risk factors can be significantly improved by an aerobic exercise program:

- Blood levels of LDL, HDL and triglycerides.
- Overweight and obesity.
- Blood pressure.
- Blood sugar level in diabetics.

People with high blood cholesterol levels respond better to both dietary changes and medication if they are exercising regularly.

Along with stopping smoking, the basics for the prevention of coronary heart disease are increasing physical exercise and altering the diet. The right diet and regular exercise will help you control your cholesterol and significantly reduce your risk of coronary heart disease.

SUMMARY

- A suitable exercise program can be prescribed at all ages.
- Before starting a program, an exercise (treadmill) test is recommended for those over 35 with coronary risk factors.
- Long, slow distance is a good way to prevent injury and get the best results from exercise.
- Exercise has a wide range of benefits to the body's metabolism of fats and glucose and can prevent not only diabetes but also cardiovascular disease.

Part IV

Coming Clean
with Prof. Ian

Before we discuss the new generation of enormously effective drugs that are increasingly being prescribed for cholesterol and triglyceride control, I'm going to show you how to increase your cardiovascular health without drugs.

24
The SAFE
Program

The most common method of unclogging the arteries is controlling risk factors as it does not involve any surgery or invasive procedures, and large studies have shown that heart attacks and strokes can be prevented at an acceptable cost to the community.

Several treatments have been shown to help reduce plaque size:
- Lifestyle changes
- Drugs to raise HDL (good cholesterol) (see Chapter 30)
- Drugs to lower LDL (bad cholesterol) (See Chapter 29)
- Surgery to lower LDL (See Chapter 33)
- Drugs to lower blood pressure

Drug therapy is not the only way to reduce plaque. Quitting smoking plus diet, exercise and anti-stress therapy are also effective.

The SAFE© Program
The SAFE program is what my team calls my hobby horse. It's my

own special invention to help my patients increase the level of their cardiovascular health.

I worked out the SAFE program over many years of treating patients with high triglycerides, who often also had other problems with their blood fats (especially low HDL). SAFE is an easily remembered acronym, and summarises the lifestyle changes that help to control triglycerides and other blood fats.

SAFE =

- Sugars
- Alcohol
- Fats
- Exercise

The SAFE program is a method of controlling triglycerides and other blood fats, often without drug treatment. If drugs are necessary, the SAFE program will greatly help to control blood fats. Let's look at the components of the program in more detail.

S=Sugars

Sugars need to be avoided in the SAFE program. Sugars are refined carbohydrates, and include:

Monosaccharides:
- glucose (in glucose-enriched drinks used typically by sportspeople)
- fructose (in fruit, fruit juices and honey)
- galactose (a component of lactose in milk)
- mannose (derived from the breakdown of plant carbohydrates)

Disaccharides:
- sucrose (in cane or table sugar, the commonest source of refined carbohydrates)

- lactose (in milk)
- maltose (in malt and germinating seeds)

During digestion, disaccharides are converted into monosaccharides:
- sucrose becomes glucose and fructose
- lactose becomes glucose and galactose
- maltose becomes glucose

The common denominator in refined carbs is therefore glucose, the sugar on which the body depends for a ready supply of energy.

Glucose can be obtained not only from food sources, but is readily manufactured by the body from protein, fats and the major source, glycogen. Glycogen is the storage form of glucose, and comprises glucose molecules joined together like links in a long chain. Glycogen is stored in tiny granules within each cell (visible by the electron microscope), especially in the liver and muscle cells that have a high rate of energy expenditure.

Blood glucose can be used in several ways after being transported into the body cells through the action of the hormone, insulin. It can be:
- Oxidised (by adding oxygen, it is converted into carbon dioxide and water), releasing energy for metabolism.
- Stored as glycogen.
- Converted into triglycerides and stored for later conversion into heat and energy for metabolism.
- Converted into proteins and other cell constituents.

Proteins and triglycerides can also be converted to glucose, so the body is a very efficient recycling depot for all of these substances.

Glucose and blood triglycerides
Some people readily convert glucose into triglycerides, which are either stored as fat droplets in the liver or secreted into the blood as VLDL particles. For this reason, people with high blood triglycerides

should reduce the intake of refined carbohydrates *from whatever source.*

Here is a list of some foods that contain these triglyceride-producing sugars:

- Cakes
- Biscuits
- Cordials
- Soft drinks
- Sweets
- Chocolates
- Honey
- Fruit (especially glace and dried fruits)
- Fruit juices (especially sweetened)
- Commercial muesli and cereals
- Liqueurs, sweet wine

Read the labels to find out how much refined carbohydrates are in a particular food. Here is the label from a typical wheat biscuit cereal:

	Per serve	Per 100g
Energy	430kJ	1200kJ
Carbohydrate	18.6g	55.8g
Sugars	0.3g	0.9g
Fibre	4.3g	12.8g
Starches	14.0g	42.1g

The table tells us:

- There are about three servings in 100g of cereal.
- The amount of sugar is quite low compared to fibre, total carbohydrate and starches, because:

Starches = (total carbohydrate) − (sugar) − (fibre)

Starches and fibre are complex carbohydrates, which are either digested less rapidly than refined carbohydrates or not digested at all. They have generally less effect on raising triglycerides and blood sugars. Non-digested carbohydrates have the important function of maintaining bowel function through providing bulk in the intestinal contents.

Compare these amounts of carbs with the typical high-sugar breakfast cereal that kids love to eat:

	Per serve	Per 100g
Energy	430kJ	1500kJ
Carbohydrate	21.0g	63.0g
Sugars	9.0g	27.0g
Fibre	3.5g	11.7g
Starches	8.5g	24.3g

This kind of cereal provides a sugar 'hit' that will rapidly raise blood glucose levels, and be followed by a rapid rise in insulin (a hormone produced by the pancreas that allows glucose to be metabolised and lowers blood sugar levels).

Some consequences of excessive intake of refined carbs include:
- Excessive triglycerides
- Increased LDL and low HDL
- Overweight and obesity
- Excessive insulin release
- The metabolic syndrome
- Diabetes
- Increased risk of cardiovascular disease
- Delayed low blood sugars after meals (with effects on mood such as irritability)

Raised triglycerides have been shown to be a marker for the subsequent development of diabetes after one or more decades.

A=Alcohol
A heavy binge-drinking session can rapidly increase triglyceride levels. If they exceed 11.0, an attack of acute pancreatitis can be precipi-

tated in susceptible people. Acute pancreatitis is a medical emergency because the following sequence of events can occur rapidly:

- Sudden release into the blood and abdominal cavity of digestive enzymes from the pancreas.
- Digestion of the body's own tissues (auto-digestion).
- Inflammation of the lining of the abdominal cavity (acute peritonitis).
- Acute, severe abdominal pain.
- A potentially fatal outcome.

Treatment of acute pancreatitis involves abstaining from alcohol, and inhibiting pancreatic secretions through intravenous feeding.

In sensitive people, even one or two glasses of alcohol a day may raise triglycerides to abnormal levels. Minimising alcohol intake is a key principle for controlling triglycerides.

Some people reduce their alcohol intake by about a half, while they also carry out the other components of the SAFE program, and see how their triglycerides respond after several weeks. If necessary they can cut back alcohol further after the next blood test.

Here are some simple ways to cut down alcohol intake:

- Change to light beer or non-alcoholic beer.
- Drink soda and bitters.
- Don't mix your drinks.
- You don't have to get drunk to enjoy yourself. Getting 'high on air' means you can have fun without the need for drugs and alcohol.
- Don't be afraid to say 'No thanks' when you are offered a drink.
- Have one or two AFD (alcohol-free days) a week.

F=Fats

Fat intake needs to be controlled in the SAFE program. Most people need to especially reduce *saturated* fats in order to lower blood triglycerides effectively. Others need to cut down on all sources of fats, whether derived from saturated, polyunsaturated or monounsaturated sources. These people usually have very high blood triglycerides (above 4.0) due to either chylomicrons or excessive VLDL.

Fish oils are the only dietary fats that don't need to be avoided, because they help lower blood triglycerides.

E=Exercise

Exercise is a critical component of the SAFE program because it has multiple beneficial effects on the body's metabolism, including blood fats: triglycerides are lowered and HDL raised.

In general, the higher the intensity of exercise and the longer the duration, the greater the changes in blood fats.

An individualised exercise program is within the province of every doctor, and should be organised according to age, muscle and joint problems, previous cardiovascular disease, and the time and motivation to perform exercise. See Chapter 23 for more.

Motivation and behaviour change

Q: How many light bulbs does it take to be a psychiatrist?

A: One, but only if you want to change.

Making changes in behaviour is one of the most difficult things for many of us to achieve. **Why?**

Because we are accustomed to repetitive behaviour patterns that cause us minimal anxiety and are easiest for us to perform. We actually prefer to act as automatons; we establish what we like to do, and we stick to it.

Changing patterns of behaviour is stressful—we have to make conscious efforts to do so, and get out of our comfort zone.

Thousands of books have been written on this topic by psychologists and all manner of people. Look at the diet books on the shelves! They are all, in a sense, books to encourage behaviour change.

So, here are a few hints on how to achieve change which may be helpful.

1. You have to understand the reasons why change is needed: *understanding is one key*.

2. You have to accept these reasons as valid: *you'll never do anything you don't believe in*.

3. You have to want to change.

4. You have to accept that the proposed changes are the best alternatives for you and that they are tailored specifically to your needs.

- Don't listen to the neighbour or your friends who tell you to do something different.
- Have ONE person directing the show (your health professional).
- Get a second opinion from an expert if you are not satisfied.
- Anything you do must be individually tailored to your needs and abilities.

5. You have to decide when to make the change, and if more than one change is needed, in what order you initiate them.

- It's hard to make more than one change at a time.
- If several changes are needed, get them into an order of priority and work on them sequentially.

6. You have to decide whether to make the changes gradually or in one step. Some people successfully stop smoking by going 'cold turkey'. Others like to reduce slowly, but often renege.

7. You have to monitor (measure) the effects of the change in terms of wellbeing and the reasons for which the change has been made.

- If you feel terrible, the changes won't work because you won't stick to them.
- Measure the things you are trying to change, but not too often (weight should be measured no more than weekly, cholesterol no more than monthly, and HDL no more than 3-monthly)

8. You have to be prepared to renege—and renegotiate.
- No-one is perfect!
- Relapses are common.
- Just get back on the rails as soon as you can.

9. You may need to start all over again.
- If this is happening time and time again, something is wrong with your strategy.
- Seek advice in this case.

10. A small change in the right direction may be enough to make the difference you need.
- Losing only 5 per cent of body weight can make a 50 per cent difference in insulin sensitivity, leading to much better control of blood fats and sugar.
- Lowering cholesterol by 1 per cent reduces heart attack risk by 1 per cent.
- Don't be disappointed if you don't get to target right away: you have already gained some benefits by moving towards them.

SUMMARY

- Most people can control triglyceride levels by modifying behaviour and lifestyle. Other blood fats will also be improved by the SAFE program.
  - S = sugars: avoid
  - A = alcohol: control
  - F = fats: control
  - E = exercise: maximise
- Changing behaviour is complex—understand the issues, make the changes, monitor what happens, and re-adjust if necessary.

25
A Seven Step Plan to Clear Arteries

Often I see patients who find they have cholesterol problems after a work-organised insurance health check. For example, Richard, a 45-year-old accountant, was found to have an elevated cholesterol level of 6.9. Let's follow his progress step by step, to see what he and his GP need to do to control his cholesterol.

Richard: a step-by-step plan to clear arteries

Richard has been well previously, with no evident risk factors other than a family history: his sister had a coronary bypass at the age of 59. She had been a heavy smoker before the bypass but Richard is not sure of her cholesterol level.

Richard weighs 95kg, his height is 185cm, his waist circumference 100cm and blood pressure 145/89mmHg.

Step 1. What is Richard's blood fat profile?

There is usually little difference between fasting and non-fasting cholesterol levels. Nevertheless, it is always necessary to confirm the high cholesterol level in case of laboratory error (a rare but potentially important factor), or other reasons.

At the same time, it is important to also measure triglycerides, HDL and LDL, and obtain a total blood fat profile.

While the fasting blood test is being done, it is a convenient time to check other causes for high cholesterol including liver, kidney and thyroid disease and diabetes. This can be done from the same blood sample.

Richard's blood fat profile is: cholesterol 6.8 (normal 4.0–6.0), triglycerides 3.3 (normal 1.0–2.0), HDL 0.8 (normal 1.0–2.0) and LDL 4.5 (normal 2.0–4.0). His other tests are normal other than a fasting glucose of 6.9 (normal less than 6.0)..

Step 2. What is his coronary risk assessment?

There is a very useful tool called the NZ Cardiovascular Risk Calculator (see Chapter 7). According to the NZ cardiovascular risk calculator, Richard has a risk of heart attack and stroke of 5–10 per cent over the next five years, based on his blood pressure, age, gender, smoking habits and diabetes status. This is at the lower range for his age, but because of the family history, it may be appropriate to increase his risk to 10–15 per cent.

Richard is at high risk of heart disease because he is aged over 45, has a significant family history, a high fasting glucose level, and has an LDL over 4. An adjusted NZ risk score of 10–15 per cent is therefore probably more appropriate. At this risk level, cholesterol-lowering drug treatment is recommended.

Using AusDiab criteria, Richard also has the metabolic syndrome (see Chapter 21):

- His systolic blood pressure is over 140mmHg.
- He has an impaired fasting glucose level (6.1–6.9).
- He has a waist circumference of 102cm or more.
- His triglycerides are above 2 and HDL below 1.

The presence of the metabolic syndrome increases Richard's risk of cardiovascular disease. Richard is told about his increased risk, and that he needs to get his risk factors under control, especially his cholesterol. A six-week period of dietary and lifestyle change is necessary and fasting blood fats including cholesterol levels will be checked again. He is advised that he may need drug treatment unless there is a significant improvement in his risk factors.

Step 3. A six-week lifestyle and dietary program

Richard sees a qualified dietitian, is given lots of advice on the right foods to buy, cook and eat, and useful hints for going out to restaurants (see Chapter 14). Best of all he gets regular support from the dietitian, has someone with whom to discuss when he 'falls off the low-chol wagon', and if there are problems it is suggested he comes to chat to me.

On this new program Richard has cut down his habitual four to five glasses of wine a day to one or two glasses. He gives away desserts, cakes, biscuits and his usual high-fat, high-sugar mid-morning and mid-afternoon snacks. Instead he eats nuts, dried fruit, low-fat ricotta and cottage cheese and other healthy snacks (see Chapter 14).

He stops eating bacon and eggs for breakfast and has porridge, fruit, low-sugar homemade muesli or baked beans on wholemeal, unbuttered or un-margarined toast. He has two or more fish meals a week. He has two vegetarian meals a week. The rest of the time he has lean chicken, lean pork, red meat with all visible fat removed or veal with a salad and one small potato instead of his usual three or four, and definitely no sour cream, when low-fat yoghurt tastes just as good.

He drinks several glasses of water a day instead of having tea or coffee with milk and sugar. He has a few egg-white omelettes for breakfast with juice, and gives the egg yolks to the dog.

Richard also walks around the block several times in the morning before breakfast and at night before bed. The dog has never looked fitter (Richard says this is because he has been getting the egg yolks, but according to his wife Susan, it's the exercise).

Even Richard has noticed a change in his waistline after three weeks on the program, but his weight hasn't shifted much.

After six weeks, Richard has lost 4kg, feels more alert, and is also sleeping better (must be stopping coffee during the day, he says, but of course the exercise helps with that too, to say nothing of not going to bed with an overloaded stomach). His waist circumference is now 97cm, and his blood pressure down to 135/85mmHg. The biggest surprises are the blood results: glucose 5.4, cholesterol 5.6, triglycerides 2.1, HDL 1.0 and LDL 3.6.

Step 4. Has his risk factor improved?
Richard's risk factor profile has improved. He no longer meets the Heart Foundation criteria for high risk, because his LDL has fallen below 4.0. According to the NZ chart, his risk has fallen to 2.5–5.0 per cent (when doubled for the family history, this comes out to 5–10 per cent), so he has gone down one risk colour.

Richard is told he does not need medication to lower cholesterol at this stage, but this will be reviewed on a six-monthly to an annual basis. Richard's doctor congratulates him but says this is the first of a series of assessments. There is a strong chance that all Richard's good intentions will weaken as the months slip by, unless he is reminded of the need to keep himself under control.

Richard is reminded of his investment: 'For every 1 per cent drop in cholesterol there is a 1 per cent fall in risk of heart attack.' He is also reminded that controlling risk factors will not only reduce his risk of future stroke, but also help prevent diabetes, slow down the progression of any plaques that may be present in the arteries, possibly induce actual regression of plaques, and help prevent new plaques from forming. He will also feel better with weight loss and more exercise.

Step 5. Modifying risk factors further
Fortunately, Richard has avoided the need for cholesterol-lowering medication at this stage. Lifestyle change is all that is necessary—but Richard has to stick to it.

Step 6. Setting long-term targets

Richard is set a realistic target for weight: 88kg (he used to be 85kg when an active sportsman many years ago). Perhaps more importantly, a waist circumference of less than 90cm is set to reduce the metabolic complications of central obesity (see Chapter 34). Richard's target blood fats are: triglycerides less than 2, LDL less than 3, HDL greater than 1, and cholesterol less than 5. These are set arbitrarily by the doctor on the basis of 'intermediate' risk between high and low.

Step 7. Richard's maintenance program

This involves continuation of lifestyle changes, with regular risk factor monitoring (usually annually if not on drug treatment, otherwise every six months). The changes begun in Step 3 are continued, often at a slightly less aggressive level depending on a number of factors such as motivation (of Richard as well as his GP), how close current risk factors are to targets, and how easily or difficult it is to stick to the program.

Generally, constant reinforcement is needed from all concerned—especially partners, friends and spouses. Self-rewards also help (Richard decides to attend that class on conversational French after all, when he gets his weight below 90kg—he is now planning an overseas holiday as a bigger reward when he reaches his blood fat targets).

Richard's doctor builds into the program a 'zone of flexibility'. He realises that Richard may stray from the job at hand, as he is a busy professional person with occasional conferences, travel, and periods of stress and strain that may make it difficult to exercise every day or avoid the extra glass of wine or two. 'If this happens, don't worry because it's easy to get back on the rails again. The important thing is to be aware of the need to get back sooner rather than later,' his doctor says.

Richard is motivated. His wife and friends help. He sees his doctor every 12 months for risk assessment and manages to achieve his goals. He has actually reduced his chance of suffering from a stroke or heart attack in the next several years by almost one-third, with even greater benefit in the longer term.

SUMMARY

- Controlling blood fats is done in the context of controlling overall (global) risk factors and assessment of coronary risk.
- Repeat fasting blood fats is necessary to confirm the abnormality.
- Underlying diseases are excluded or treated.
- A fairly aggressive short-term program is followed by a maintenance program that may or may not include drug treatment.
- Aim for 5 per cent lower body weight to start with—this will improve the body's handling of cholesterol and triglycerides as well as lowering blood pressure.
- Eat low-salt products. Don't add salt at the table or in cooking (your palate will soon get used to the low-salt cuisine and you'll notice bread is usually very salty and celery is almost inedible because it tastes too salty.
- Cut back alcohol to two standard drinks a day or less (alcohol raises blood pressure).
- Lower your intake of saturated (animal) fats—this will help lower blood pressure.
- Increase your exercise levels; this not only helps lose weight, but also helps the blood vessels relax and lowers blood pressure.
- Medications may be necessary for some people, but don't start them until you have tried all of the above methods (unless your blood pressure is dangerously high, when medications may be necessary from the start).
- Lowering blood pressure and lowering cholesterol and triglycerides work together to lower the risk of heart attack and stroke.

26
How Low Do You Go?

A term which is relatively new in modern medical practice is *evidence-based* medicine.

This means exactly what it says: the results of the latest research are, on evidence, incorporated into recommendations for treatment. Once we have the evidence we can initiate the appropriate regimens or programs. These are constantly being updated—therefore 'changing the goalposts' is something both doctors and the general public have to be aware of, be prepared to adapt to, and accept.

Sometimes the latest evidence contradicts earlier evidence and the goalposts change yet again—very frustrating for doctors and patients alike. Some people take the easy option and say, 'They can never make up their minds. I'll stick to what I used to do!' This is a head-in-the-sand attitude, and if we were to adopt such a philosophy, we'd still be living in caves, hunting for our dinners and wearing animal skins!

As evidence accumulates, and one trial is confirmed by another, and yet another, the point is reached where there is no longer any argument. This process may take years or even generations, depending on how actively the research takes place. Knowledge in finding the best ways to unclog the arteries and control cholesterol and triglycerides is no different, except that research in these areas is so intense that, inevitably, certain recommendations for treatment change as often as every two or three years.

In this chapter, we'll discuss where the latest goalposts lie.

As I said in one of my previous book, *Men's Health*: 'You cannot fight an unknown enemy.' To combat heart attack and stroke—the biggest killers in our societies—we have to take every advantage we can. Knowledge is a key to preventative action.

We need to be aware of the current recommendations for LDL, HDL and triglycerides. Then we can consider these levels with greater understanding, and be motivated to achieve better results. In general, people at high risk need to achieve lower cholesterol, LDL and triglycerides, and aim for higher levels of HDL.

Recommended LDL levels

For those at high risk for heart attack and stroke, LDL should be less than 2.0. People at high risk are those with:

1. Existing vascular disease
   - After heart attack, coronary bypass surgery or coronary angioplasty/stenting (see Chapter 34).
   - Those with chest pain or heart failure due to clogging of the coronary arteries.
   - After stroke or transient ischaemic attacks.
   - Those with arterial disease of the abdominal aorta or legs.
2. Diabetes
3. Chronic kidney disease
4. Familial hypercholesterolaemia
5. Aboriginal or Torres Strait Islander origin
6. 15 per cent or more risk of cardiovascular disease in the next five years, as determined by the New Zealand Risk Calculator Chart (see Chapter 7).
7. 10–15 per cent risk of cardiovascular disease in the next five years in the presence of any of the following:

- First degree relatives with coronary disease before age 60.
- The metabolic syndrome (see Chapter 21).

A lower recommended LDL of 1.8 was recently made in the US for people who have had a recent heart attack (see Chapter 38).

Recommended HDL levels

The recommended HDL for those at high risk is greater than 1.0. The evidence for this is not based on clinical trials as for LDL, but rather on population studies and other scientific evidence. The American Diabetes Association recommends higher HDL levels in diabetic women than diabetic men (1.2 vs. 1.0).

Recommended triglyceride levels

The recommended level for triglycerides for those at high risk is less than 1.5. As for HDL, there are no trials specifically designed to lower only triglycerides, but there is a large amount of scientific evidence from population and other studies to suggest this recommendation.

Other recommendations for diabetics

The American Diabetes Association has another special recommendation for diabetics with high triglycerides above 4.5, when it is not reliable to measure LDL. The special recommendation is for the non-HDL level to be 3.5 or less. For example, let's look at a diabetic person with the following blood fats:

    Cholesterol   6.5
    Triglycerides   6.6
    HDL   0.5
    (LDL cannot be calculated because triglycerides are greater
        than 4.5)

The level of non-HDL for this person is 6.5–0.5 = 6.0, well above the ADA target of 3.5.

Recommendations for people at intermediate risk of heart attack or stroke

These are people who are at potentially high risk, but do not meet the above criteria for high risk, and have one or more of the following risk factors:

- Cigarette smoking
- Family history of coronary heart disease (first degree relative affected before the age of 60)
- Overweight, especially the metabolic syndrome
- High blood pressure
- Impaired glucose tolerance or raised fasting blood glucose level
- Impaired kidney function (blood creatinine level 0.13 or above) or micro-albuminuria (the presence of albumin in the urine that is insufficient to be detected by dip-sticks)
- Age 45+
- HDL less than 1.0
- People who have a 10–15 per cent or more cardiovascular risk according to the New Zealand Core Committee risk factor chart

Recommended LDL for this intermediate-risk group is less than 3.4 according to current US and European guidelines. In view of recent trial results, however, a lower LDL target of less than 3.0 is more appropriate.

Recommendations for people at low risk of heart attack and stroke

Low-risk people are not in any of the above groups. The recommended LDL is less than 3.8 according to current European and US guidelines, but because lower LDL targets for other risk categories are now recommended, it is appropriate to also recommend lower LDL less than 3.4 for those with low risk.

SUMMARY

- Recommended levels for people at high risk of heart attack and stroke are:
- LDL less than 2.0
- Triglycerides less than 1.5
- HDL greater than 1.0
- It is important to realise that, although recommended levels are not achieved, there is considerable benefit from any lowering of LDL.
- Remember, 1 per cent reduction in LDL translates into 1 per cent lower risk of heart attack risk.
- 1 per cent higher HDL also translates into a 1 per cent lower heart attack risk.

27

Success Stories
From My Casebook

I often think I have learnt as much from my patients as they have learnt from me. Certainly they have all been very generous in allowing me to talk about their cases and to use their treatment as role models for teaching purposes. Wayne whom I have been looking after for some time, loves to hear that I have told his success story.

WAYNE: OVERFED, UNDER-EXERCISED AND OVERWEIGHT

Wayne is a 40-year-old sales executive for a city department store. He is a non-smoker. He has no family history of coronary heart disease. His parents are alive and well, in their seventies. He is one of two brothers, and has two healthy children.

Since his marriage 20 years ago, he has given up playing regular sport, and does not do any regular exercise. He drinks one or two glasses of wine a day on average, and two or three schooners of beer on weekends over the summer.

He eats three meals a day, and usually has a biscuit or slice of cake for afternoon tea and supper. Breakfast consists of a glass of orange juice, cup of white coffee with sugar, two slices of white toast with butter and jam, and sometimes he has poached, boiled or scrambled eggs. On weekends he cooks eggs and bacon for the family breakfast. He always has a light lunch (a sandwich, usually beef and horseradish or sometimes a pie or pasty) and drinks several cups of tea (white, one sugar) during the working day.

He feels that he is coping with work without being aware of stress or pressure. His home life is happy, his sexual activity normal, and he sleeps soundly eight hours a night. He does not take drugs, minerals or vitamin supplements.

He arrives home from work at about 6pm, watches the news on television, then reads the evening paper while his wife prepares the dinner and his children finish off their homework.

For dinner, he will usually have no entree or soup, but start with the main meal. He prefers roast beef, roast lamb, steak and chips to most foods, and usually has a serve of buttered vegetables with his meat. He has two slices of white bread with butter. For dessert, he has usually ice-cream in summer, often with chocolate topping. In winter he often has a cake-based hot pudding with custard (made from the same packet). He finishes off the meal with another cup of coffee, and settles down to watch the evening's television—with a bowl of nuts and sweets, and perhaps later a hot drink and sweet biscuits.

Wayne looks well. He is 174cm tall and weighs 79kg. His fasting blood fat profile is: cholesterol 6.3 (normal 4.0-6.0), HDL 1.0 (normal 1.0-2.0), triglycerides 1.4 (normal 1.0-2.0) and LDL 4.7 (normal 2.0-4.0). His blood pressure is normal at 140/85 mmHg.

According to the New Zealand risk factor assessment chart, he is at low risk for heart attack and stroke—approximately 2.5–5 per cent in the next five years. This risk can be reduced to less than 2.5 per cent by lowering his cholesterol or raising his HDL (see Chapter 7). At this low level of risk, he does not need medication to lower his cholesterol.

I explain the reasons for Wayne's high blood cholesterol level:

- 'Your ideal body weight for your height and age is 72kg. Your present weight is 7kg over this, which is 10 per cent above ideal body weight.
- 'You have a sedentary lifestyle (at least, after your marriage to Sandra 20 years ago).
- 'You eat too many *empty calories* in the form of alcohol and sugar (these are high-energy foods that have relatively little protein, fat, complex carbohydrates, vitamins and minerals—in other words, very little nutritive value apart from energy).
- 'You need to lower your cholesterol. Fortunately, you have no other risk factors: you have no family history of coronary heart disease, you are a non-smoker, have normal blood pressure and are otherwise generally well. This means your risk score will fall considerably after you lower your cholesterol.
- 'You eat too much cholesterol (about 600 mg per day) and total fat (40 per cent of your daily energy is provided by fat). You have a high intake of saturated fats with a relatively low intake of polyunsaturated fats and monounsaturated fats. Your ratio of polyunsaturated fats to saturated fats is low (about 0.5).
- 'Further detailed analysis of your diet shows a high energy intake. You are not deficient in any particular vitamin or mineral. You have a high intake of refined carbohydrates (simple sugars) and a low intake of complex carbohydrates and fibre.'

Wayne's treatment plan is to discuss the factors leading to his blood cholesterol problem, and to give advice on modifying his lifestyle in the following way:

- Wayne is asked to choose a form of exercise that he enjoys. Some people prefer walking, others bicycling, others swimming. Most younger people can take on a not-too-strenuous mix of walking and jogging which they can gradually build up. Because exercises that improve cardiac and respiratory fitness—'aerobic' activity—are preferred, weight-lifting is not recommended.

- He is warned that he may get short of breath very quickly, get dry in the mouth and have the experience of dryness in his throat and upper lungs because of the unaccustomed increased respiratory activity. He may also experience palpitations—awareness of the heartbeat. He may also sweat readily. All of these are normal in the unfit beginner undertaking mild exercise, and become much less noticeable with increasing fitness.

- Wayne is advised not to jog or run on the footpath or road as this, especially in the unfit and overweight, places unaccustomed strain on the joints and ligaments, particularly of the ankles, knees and hips. Wayne is advised to jog or run on grass, which is much softer on the bones and joints.

- Wayne is reminded of the importance of stretching his legs and arms before starting off on his morning walk or jog. Have you seen how the cat and dog give themselves a good stretch before they run off to their breakfast bowls?

Having chosen a mixture of walking and jogging, Wayne decides what times of the day best suit him to start his exercise program. He decides on the early morning before breakfast: 7 to 7.30am. He buys a good pair of jogging shoes, including synthetic foam-rubber shock-absorbing inner soles, and finds his old football shorts in the bottom drawer of the wardrobe. Wayne begins with a walk to the local park, a distance of 500 metres, then jogs slowly around (which takes five minutes) once every day.

Wayne's consumption of empty calories has to stop. He is firmly advised to stop using sugar of any form. Sugar has been called 'sweet, white and deadly'. Sugar in the diet is unnecessary; Wayne's body makes it when required, and sugar in the diet provides too many calories that he is storing away as body fat.

Wayne also needs to cut down his alcohol to no more than one glass of wine a day, and two glasses of low-alcohol beer a weekend. Depending on his progress, Wayne may be advised to stop alcohol altogether, and use alcohol substitutes: Birrell (a Swiss brewed-in-the-bottle ale with almost no alcohol content, which is very like the real thing but a bit sweeter) instead of beer, Claytons for aperitifs and cocktails, and the excellent all-round non-alcoholic long drink, iced soda and bitters, with a slice of lemon.

Wayne's cholesterol intake of 500 mg/day is way over the recommended level of 300 mg/day. There are three main sources of cholesterol in his diet: egg yolks (250 mg of cholesterol per yolk), dairy products (milk, ice-cream, cream, cheese and butter) and meat.

Wayne is advised to stop eating egg yolks altogether—they are unnecessary and provide concentrated cholesterol. He is advised to stop eating his usual dairy products. Cream is forbidden, as is whole milk and butter.

Polyunsaturated margarine is not recommended in place of butter because both butter and margarine are very high in calories. Instead, Wayne is advised to do without butter or margarine on his bread.

Wayne's total fat intake is also high: he should have less than 30 per cent of total energy from fats and at present has 40 per cent. He should have less than 10 per cent of his total energy from saturated fat, and the dietary ratio of saturated to polyunsaturated fats should be about 1:1. At present, for every 1 g of polyunsaturated fat, he is eating 2 g of saturated fat.

Rather than increasing Wayne's polyunsaturated fat intake (which will increase his calories) he is advised to cut down on saturated fats. Because saturated fats occur with cholesterol, the ways to cut down on cholesterol intake also cut down on saturated fat intake. Wayne therefore avoids full-cream dairy products. He also cuts off any visible fat from his meat, and has nothing cooked in fat (either deep-fried or pan-fried).

In these days of the microwave revolution and pan-liners, fat-free cooking is very straightforward and simple. Fat (of any kind, whether animal or vegetable) has the highest energy value of any foods—about 9kcal/g, compared with about 4kcal/g for protein and carbohydrates. For weight loss, 'fats make fat' should be the motto.

Wayne is advised to eat more fruit, wholemeal bread, high-fibre cereals, and to stop eating jam, honey and any high-sugar food, such as biscuits and cake (which also have a high saturated fat content). He is referred to a qualified dietitian for more advice.

Wayne comes back every two weeks to check progress. After eight weeks on his program, he has lost 6kg in weight and his blood cholesterol level is 5.4. Wayne has done well.

Since losing weight and lowering his blood cholesterol, Wayne feels ten years younger and describes himself as 'dangerous'—his sexual activity has increased, his mental concentration improved, and he is enjoying work and leisure more than before. Now Wayne's goal is to continue his program.

Wayne returns in six months for a re-check of his blood cholesterol levels—and to see how he is going.

MARK: ALCOHOL-INDUCED HIGH BLOOD CHOLESTEROL

Mark is a 30-year-old journalist who works for a large city newspaper. For the last five years he has not smoked, although he smoked 30 cigarettes a day during the previous five years. He has no known family history of coronary heart disease. He is single and enjoys an active social life. He goes out to dine at least three times a week, and often is invited to friends' parties. He isn't in a steady relationship, and feels unsure about whether he is ready to 'settle down'.

He lives alone in a flat in a trendy part of the city. He doesn't usually eat breakfast, arriving at work a little after 9 in the morning. At 10am he goes across the road to the local snack bar and orders black coffee with two sugars and a toasted egg-and-bacon sandwich. While waiting for his brunch he reads the previous evening's newspaper and checks his daily schedule. At lunchtime he often goes to the local pub with his workmates and often meets friends there. For lunch he normally has a steak and mixed vegetables, with several glasses of red wine. During the afternoon he has two more cups of black coffee, each with two sugars.

Twice a week after work he plays tennis with friends. During the evening he drinks several large glasses of beer and eats several packets of potato chips and nuts. After the game he often invites a friend home, has several more glasses of wine over the evening and eats supper at about 11pm, usually scrambled eggs or an omelette.

On examination, Mark looks fit, although somewhat dissipated. He is 185cm tall, and weighs 86kg. His ideal body weight is 74kg, so that he is 16 per cent above ideal body weight. His systolic blood pressure is high at 172 mmHg (normal less than 140), with a normal pulse rate of 70 beats per minute. There are no other abnormal physical findings.

Mark's fasting blood fat profile is: cholesterol 8.6 (normal 4-6), HDL 0.7 (normal 1.0-2.0), triglycerides 6.8 (normal 1.0-2.0), LDL unable to calculate because triglycerides over 4.5. According to the risk factor assessment chart, Mark has a very high coronary risk score of 87 (high risk for his age is above 34).

Mark's doctor explains the reasons for Mark's high cholesterol and blood pressure:

- 'You're drinking an average of six glasses of wine and six glasses of beer per day; wine contains about 10 per cent and beer about 5 per cent alcohol, giving a daily alcohol intake of about 120 g. Recent studies have shown that an alcohol intake in excess of 60 g per day may result in fatty degeneration of the liver, leading to cirrhosis of the liver and eventually to liver failure.

- 'Your current level of alcohol intake also is likely to cause progressive damage to your brain cells, pancreas, stomach and intestine.

- 'Your high blood pressure is also aggravated by your

alcohol intake: many studies have shown that alcohol intake is directly correlated to the development of high blood pressure.

- 'Finally, your high cholesterol may be caused by your high alcohol intake, because in some people alcohol alters the metabolism of the liver.'

His dietitian says: 'You have a high intake of cholesterol (600 mg per day) and saturated fat, with a dietary polyunsaturated to saturated fat ratio of about 0.4.'

Mark is advised to stop drinking alcohol for a three-week period, and to reduce his saturated fat and cholesterol intake. The dietary advice and pamphlets given to Wayne are also given to Mark, and the same books are recommended.

Four weeks later, Mark returns for a check-up. He has managed to reduce alcohol to one or two glasses of wine a day and has stopped drinking beer all together. He has lost 4kg in weight and feels generally better. His blood cholesterol level has fallen to 6.1, his HDL level increased to 1.0 and triglycerides have also fallen to 3.9.

Mark is encouraged to continue the same diet and exercise program, with alcohol restricted to one glass of wine per day. Six months later he has lost another 4kg, and blood levels are: cholesterol 5.9, HDL 1.2, and triglycerides 2.1.

Three months later, his blood cholesterol level is much the same. He is advised to stop drinking alcohol altogether, and three weeks later his blood cholesterol level is 5.4, with HDL 1.3 and triglycerides 1.9.

JUDITH: LOW THYROID ACTIVITY

Judith is a 55-year-old business executive. She is a non-smoker and has no family history of coronary heart disease. Her sister, aged 65, had an overactive thyroid gland 30 years ago and is now taking medication for her thyroid gland. Judith's only symptom is that she tires easily. On examination, she is 160cm tall, weighs 70kg, and her systolic blood pressure is normal at 140mmHg. Physical examination is unremarkable except that her skin seems thinned and slightly pale and she has thin hair.

Her blood fat profile is: cholesterol 10.8 (normal 4.0–6.0), HDL 1.2 (normal 1.0–2.0), triglycerides 3.2 (normal 1.0–2.0) and LDL 8.1 (normal 2.0–4.0).

Judith is sent to the laboratory to have another blood test to check underlying causes for her high cholesterol level. The thyroid function test result shows that the thyroid is working at about half normal capacity. Further tests demonstrate that she has developed antibodies to her own thyroid gland and it seems that her thyroid problem has been of gradual onset over the preceding several years.

Judith is treated with thyroid hormone tablets. Six months later, her activity level has increased, she feels more alert and no longer tires easily. Her fasting blood fat profile is: cholesterol 4.8, HDL 1.8, triglycerides 1.4 and LDL 2.4. Judith will need to continue thyroid tablets for the rest of her life, with regular adjustments of her dose according to blood tests of her thyroid function. As long as she continues to do this, her cholesterol level will be controlled, unless other causes for high cholesterol develop.

As a result of Judith's tests, her other sister, Ruth, had her thyroid function checked and was also found to have borderline low thyroid activity. Ruth's blood cholesterol is also high at 6.9. Thyroid replacement with a low dose of thyroid hormone results in both a normal thyroid activity and an acceptable blood cholesterol level of 5.4.

ROBERT: EXTREMELY HIGH TRIGLYCERIDES

Robert is a publican. When tested by his general practitioner, he was found to have the following fasting blood fat profile after nothing to eat or drink for at least 12 hours before the test: cholesterol 22.4 (normal 4.0–6.0), triglycerides 48.6 (normal 1.0–2.0), HDL 0.4 (normal 1.0–2.0) and LDL unable to calculate.

Robert admitted to drinking 12 stubbies of beer on an average working day, sometimes as much as 20. Interspersed were a few glasses of red or white wine and the occasional scotch.

His doctor noted that Robert was at least 20kg overweight (he weighed 95kg and was 175cm in height). There was no other abnormality other than a blood pressure of 160/85 (normal blood pressure 140/80). Robert's liver function tests showed a high level of an enzyme that is raised by alcohol.

Robert was advised that his triglycerides were at a dangerous level, because he was at risk of *acute pancreatitis*. This is a disease in which the pancreas becomes acutely inflamed, and pancreatic enzymes (which dissolve fats, carbohydrates and proteins) are released into the bloodstream and the abdominal cavity, causing even more severe and widespread inflammation, and possibly death.

The goal of treatment was to reduce blood triglycerides below 11. To do this, Robert was advised to stop drinking alcohol completely, to avoid any dietary fats (whether saturated, monounsaturated or polyunsaturated), and to start taking fenofibrate to lower his triglycerides. One month later, Robert had a repeat blood fat profile: cholesterol 5.4, triglycerides 2.2, HDL 1.0 and LDL 3.4.

His liver enzymes had dropped to normal and he felt very well, although he missed his beer! The plan was then to allow Robert the occasional drink (up to four stubbies of light beer per day), liberalise his fat intake (other than avoiding saturated fats), and to continue treatment with fenofibrate.

In the longer term, Robert's aim was to lose at least 10kg in the next five months. He was referred to a dietitian for more specific advice on weight loss, and also given an exercise program.

Comments

Robert's blood fat profile is an uncommon but alarming one, with grossly elevated triglycerides and cholesterol levels, as well as a very low HDL. Surprisingly, this profile is not usually associated with increased risk for cardiovascular disease. The lipoprotein particles in the blood are very large and rich in triglycerides, and do not appear to have a great effect on atherosclerosis, possibly because they are unable to cross into the arterial wall from the blood unlike small particles such as LDL.

The danger of triglycerides above 11 is acute pancreatitis, and urgent measures are needed to control triglycerides. For this reason, Robert was started at once on fenofibrate, even though it was obvious that alcohol was the likely culprit. He was also told to avoid dietary fats, which are converted by the intestine into large triglyceride-rich particles called *chylomicrons*. If present in sufficient quantities, these particles can cause acute pancreatitis, and their formation is abolished by withholding the usual kinds of fats from the diet.

There are some people with inherited disorders of triglycerides metabolism with similar profiles to Robert's, even though they do not drink alcohol. Chylomicrons and large triglycerides-rich particles called VLDL accumulate because of a deficiency of the enzyme *lipoprotein lipase* or its cofactor *apoC-III*. They are also at risk of acute pancreatitis, and must avoid dietary fats, which can be converted into chylomicrons. Instead, *medium-chain triglycerides* derived from coconut oil can be eaten. These are triglycerides with medium-length saturated fatty acids (8–10 carbon units) which are absorbed into the blood from the intestine directly, without being packaged into chylomicrons.

Occasionally, people with angina have developed very high blood triglycerides because of alcohol excess, or other conditions such as diabetes. The symptoms of angina in these people were controlled only when their triglycerides were brought near the normal range, suggesting that very high triglycerides may interfere with the blood circulation and supply of oxygen and other nutrients to heart muscle.

JANE: GENETIC HIGH TRIGLYCERIDES

Jane went to her general practitioner because of a family history of early heart attacks, affecting several of her uncles and aunts on both sides of the family, although most were in their late sixties or early seventies at the time. The GP could find no particular problems with normal physical examination and sent Jane off for a blood fat profile.

The results were: cholesterol 8.0 (normal 4.0–6.0), triglycerides 8.4 (normal 1.0–2.0), HDL 0.8 (normal 1.0–2.0) and LDL unable to calculate.

Jane was found to have slightly low thyroid activity in another blood test, and an abnormal genetic pattern in her apoE protein. She was treated with thyroid hormone tablets, a cholesterol-lowering diet, and fenofibrate. Two months later, her blood fat profile and thyroid function had returned to normal.

Comments

It is unusual to have similar levels of triglycerides and cholesterol in a fasting blood sample—this result suggests a genetic abnormality in the apoE protein. The 2/2 gene profile is present in about one in 100 of the population but only about 1 per cent of these have high triglycerides and cholesterol levels. It is believed that another abnormality must be present in addition to the underlying genetic profile, such as low thyroid activity, diabetes, or diseases of the liver or kidneys.

When blood triglycerides are high, and due to apoE 2/2 pattern, they can be deposited in the skin creases of the palms, causing yellow-orange discolouration (*palmar xanthomas*). Other yellow fatty deposits can also occur in other areas of the skin, such as the elbows, buttocks, or the back. These can look like little raised yellow pimple-like lesions with reddened edges (*eruptive xanthomas*) or larger yellow lumpy deposits (*tuberous xanthomas*).

People with the apoE 2/2 disorder have an increased risk of clogging of the coronary arteries (causing angina and heart attack) as well as of the arteries to the legs, which may cause pain in the calves when walking (*claudication*).

SUSAN: DIABETIC

In her mid-forties, Susan decided to have a diabetes test because her mother had recently been diagnosed with mild diabetes, and had managed to control her blood glucose levels with a modified diet. Susan had a fasting blood glucose level just above the normal range and went on to have a glucose tolerance test, in which the fasting blood glucose levels were measured before and two hours after a glucose drink. The two-hour level was 12.8 (a level above 11 indicates diabetes).

Since then, Susan has been on a diabetic diet, with good control of her blood glucose levels.

Her blood fats have not been so well-controlled and at last count were: cholesterol 6.5 (normal 4.0–6.0), triglycerides 4.4 (normal 1.0–2.0), HDL 0.8 (normal 1.0–2.0) and LDL 3.7 (normal 2.0–4.0). Susan's doctor started her on fenofibrate treatment. Three months later, her blood fats were: cholesterol 6.2, triglycerides 1.8 HDL 1.0 and LDL 4.4.

Susan's doctor was puzzled. There was a definite improvement in triglycerides and slight improvement in cholesterol and HDL, but the LDL had risen. He was not happy with this profile and changed Susan to a statin at a dose of 20 mg daily. Three months later her results were: cholesterol 5.0, triglycerides 2.9, HDL 0.9 and LDL 2.8.

Once again, Susan's doctor was not completely happy with the result because of the low HDL (he wanted to see it over 1.0). The triglycerides and LDL were still a bit high. He asked for specialist advice.

The specialist explained that only fine-tuning was needed. There was a choice of either using higher doses of a statin (40 or 80 mg, depending on the response to 40 mg), or using combination drug therapy (statin plus fenofibrate, or fish oils plus statin plus fenofibrate). It was decided to increase the dose of statin to 40 mg with the following results: cholesterol 4.2, triglycerides 2.1, HDL 0.8 and LDL 2.4.

Once again the blood fat profile, while improved in some respects, was not ideal in that HDL remained low and triglycerides slightly high. Fenofibrate was added to the statin 40 mg, and at last satisfactory results were obtained: cholesterol 4.0, triglycerides 1.6, HDL 1.1 and LDL 2.2.

Comments

Susan illustrates the difficulty in achieving ideal blood fats in many people who have incomplete responses to therapy with one drug. Sometimes it is simply a matter of increasing the statin dose gradually, and sometimes statins and fenofibrate are used in combination. Some people require three or even four different drugs.

The American Diabetes Association suggests that control of LDL is the first priority in diabetics, followed by control of HDL and then triglycerides. Statin treatment is suggested as first-line, then fibrates (such as fenofibrate).

BILL: HEART ATTACK

Bill, a farmer, had a mild and uncomplicated heart attack about seven years ago. Because his cholesterol was 6.7, he was started on a statin (20 mg daily), aspirin (100 mg daily) to reduce the clotting tendency of the blood (and the risk of another heart attack) and a beta-blocker (metoprolol 50 mg daily) to slow down the heart rate and also reduce the risk of another heart attack. Since then he has been well and has made, as far as he can tell, a complete recovery.

Bill had his six-monthly check-up and was found to have the following blood fat profile: cholesterol 4.8 (normal 4.0–6.0), triglycerides 2.2 (normal 1.0–2.0), HDL 0.9 (normal 1.0–2.0) and LDL 2.9 (normal 2.0–4.0). Bill's doctor increased his dose of statin to 40 mg daily, advised Bill to tighten up his cholesterol-lowering diet, lose some weight and do more exercise. Three months later Bill had lost 4kg in weight, and a re-check of his blood fats showed: cholesterol 3.4, triglycerides 1.4, HDL 1.0 and LDL 1.8.

Bill was congratulated and advised to continue his current treatment program.

Comments

Bill's response to 20 mg dose of statin was good, but not quite good enough to meet current recommendations, which suggest the following targets for people at high risk for heart attack and stroke who require drug therapy to lower blood fat levels:

- Triglycerides less than 1.5
- HDL greater than 1.0
- LDL less than 2.0

SUMMARY

- The causes of high blood fats may be genetic or environmental, or caused by underlying diseases.
- Lifestyle changes will often make a significant improvement but drugs may also be needed.
- Testing for and treating any disease that causes high cholesterol or triglycerides is essential.

Part V

The Magic of
Modern Medicine

My patients often ask for a medication that
will unclog their arteries—a kind of 'drain-
cleaner' for the body. Modern medications do
just that—they can improve or even prevent
clogging of the arteries.

28

Medication — Oldies But Goodies

Not too many years ago, it was much easier to treat high blood pressure than high cholesterol because there was a greater range of effective medications for blood pressure whereas the drugs to lower cholesterol weren't so effective. All this changed with the advent of statins (see Chapter 29) and other drugs to control blood fats. Let's return to the good old days. The medications we used to use on a daily basis are still available to us but we now use them in more limited circumstances, and less often. In this chapter, I'll describe these medications and where they fit into current treatment.

Resins

Resins are non-absorbable powders that bind to bile acids in the intestine and prevent their absorption. For this reason they are also called bile acid sequesterants and include the medications cholestyramine and colestipol.

These medications are available in little sachets with 4 g or 5 g of active ingredients. They are insoluble in water and must be suspended in water or fruit juice. They also have a granular or gritty consistency (some people liken them to drinking sand). For these reasons alone, resins are not easy to take and many people have trouble sticking to the prescribed amounts. Resins can also cause constipation in higher doses, especially in the elderly.

Resins can lower LDL by up to 20 per cent when taken in maximum doses. An early clinical trial of maximum doses of cholestyramine lowered the heart attack rate by almost 20 per cent over a seven-year period. Published in 1984, it was one of the first trials to test the cholesterol hypothesis: that lowering cholesterol levels would reduce heart attack rates.

Resins may cause unpleasant side effects, mainly confined to the intestinal tract, including nausea, reflux, abdominal boating, flatulence and constipation, especially in high doses. One or two packets a day is about the most people can manage, especially the elderly. They are also relatively inconvenient to take, having to be mixed with liquid first.

Resins are useful for the treatment of bile acid-induced diarrhoea, as bile acids stimulate bowel contraction and are rendered less active when bound to resins.

Resins are currently used:
- In combination therapy with statins, although resins can be used with any other medications to lower LDL.
- For bile acid-induced diarrhoea.
- In children with familial hypercholesterolaemia who are too young to be given statins, or who have side effects from statins. Resins in low doses are safe because they are not absorbed and do not affect fat soluble vitamin levels. High doses, however, can result in fat soluble vitamin deficiency in children.

New resins are now available in tablet form, overcoming many of the problems with older ones; they may start to become popular again (see Chapter 30 on new medications).

Fibrates

Fibrates are used to lower triglycerides and have a variable effect on LDL (LDL may either be unaltered, lowered slightly or increased slightly, depending on the clinical situation). Fibrates also have a modest effect in raising HDL levels.

These days, they are mainly used to treat patients with high triglycerides and low HDL, usually those with either diabetes or the metabolic syndrome. Fenofibrate is often used in combination with statins.

Nicotinic acid

Nicotinic acid (also called niacin or vitamin B3) is a B vitamin required in amounts of about 25 mg daily to maintain normal health. It occurs naturally in wholegrain cereals and many other plant products.

In mega-doses of 500–3000g daily, nicotinic acid benefits blood fats; it raises HDL and lowers LDL, cholesterol and triglycerides. Nicotinic acid is currently the most powerful medication to raise HDL (up to 30 per cent).

The main problem with nicotinic acid is its tendency to cause skin flushing and irritation soon after taking the dose. Not everyone is affected to the same extent, and this side effect tends to become less pronounced with time. Rapid absorption of nicotinic acid and high blood levels are the main factors that cause the skin flushing. This depends on the rate of intestinal mobility, so nicotinic acid is always taken on a full stomach, in order to minimise the rate of absorption, and three times or twice daily to minimise high blood levels.

A new medication has recently been developed to minimise skin flushing with nicotinic acid (see Chapter 30 on new medications).

Other less common side effects include indigestion, activation of stomach ulcers, bleeding from active stomach ulcers, low blood pressure, increased blood glucose levels in diabetics, and increased liver enzymes indicating variable degrees of liver cell injury.

An extended-release tablet is available in the US, and may become available in Australia.

Nicotinic acid has been shown to reduce the rate of heart attacks in two clinical trials: one in combination with a fibrate (clofibrate) in Scandinavian men, the other in the US.

Aspirin

Some time ago a good friend of mine—a man in his late seventies—rang me late at night to complain of severe chest pain that sounded very much like the symptoms of a heart attack. He lived out in the country and fifteen minutes from the nearest town. My advice was simple: 'First of all, ring the ambulance. While you do that, ask your wife to get an aspirin tablet, chew it up, and swallow it with a bit of water. Sit quietly and relax as much as possible until the ambulance comes, when you'll be in good hands. They'll take you to the nearest emergency department. I'll give them a call to tell them you're on the way.'

Peter did have a heart attack—his first—and survived to tell the story. He actually went on to have an angiogram, an angioplasty and a stent, but that's not the purpose of this story. The evidence is that aspirin's rapid action as an anti-clotting agent helped keep Peter's artery sufficiently unclogged for it to beat strongly and normally in the first hour or so of his attack, and to survive it with minimal damage to his heart muscle. A dose of at least 162 mg daily should be used in the event of a heart attack (one standard tablet is 300 mg).

In fact, for certain people aspirin has been the cheapest and most cost-effective medication to prevent heart disease and stroke.

What are the risks of aspirin treatment?

Firstly, because aspirin is an anti-clotting agent, there is a slightly increased risk of bleeding. Anyone who has taken an aspirin (for a headache or fever) will have noticed that it takes much longer for a cut to stop bleeding for a few days afterwards. The anti-clotting effects of aspirin actually last for about five days. This is because there is a constant turnover of the cells (called platelets) that are affected by aspirin. When the bone marrow has produced enough new platelets, the bleeding time returns to normal.

The increased bleeding tendency is a nuisance in most people (for example, after a cut), but for a minority can be serious. There is a tiny but significant risk (when all the millions of people on aspirin are taken into consideration) of a stroke caused by cerebral haemorrhage. Those with genetic clotting tendencies are also at risk of increased bleeding if they take aspirin. The most common site for bleeding is, however, from the bowel. Aspirin significantly increased 'occult' (hidden) bleeding, which cannot be detected visually. In those with previous intestinal bleeding, the amount of occult bleeding may be enough to cause anaemia (low levels of red blood cells). This, in turn, can result in a low oxygen-carrying capacity of the blood, with shortness of breath and fatigue on exercise.

Aspirin is also a stomach irritant. It can actually increase the risk of stomach and duodenal ulcers, as well as bleeding from these ulcers, which may be dangerous. For these reasons, aspirin is often taken in an 'enteric-coated' form, when the tablet has a coating to prevent release of aspirin in the stomach. This kind of aspirin has a lower risk of stomach irritation (but it is still greater than if aspirin were not taken).

Aspirin can uncommonly cause skin rashes and asthma due to allergy. So like any other drug, there are pros and cons on aspirin's balance sheet. Overall, aspirin is highly effective to prevent recurrent heart attacks and strokes (i.e. in the setting of secondary prevention). A daily dose of 75–100 mg is required for effective anti-clotting activity. This compares with the dose of aspirin for pain or fever relief of up to 300 mg two to four times daily in adults (smaller doses are used for kids).

In the setting of primary prevention, aspirin is currently used for people at high risk for heart attack and stroke (this is especially the case for diabetics and, some believe, the elderly).

SUMMARY

- Resins, fibrates and nicotinic acid are the 'old favourites' whose use has largely been superceded by statins.
- These drugs are still useful for some people, and can be very effective in controlling cholesterol and triglycerides when used appropriately.
- Aspirin is the oldest 'wonder drug' and effectively reduces risk of heart attack and stroke, especially in those who've previously suffered such events.
- Anybody taking aspirin for the first time must review any history of a bleeding tendency (is there a genetic basis for this?), intestinal problems (have they had a stomach or duodenal ulcer?), asthma (are they allergic to aspirin?) and previous cardiovascular disease.
- It's dangerous, as one would expect, to treat a person who has had a previous cerebral haemorrhage or bleeding tendency with aspirin.
- In contrast, people who have had the usual form of stroke (due to a cerebral infarct) require aspirin to reduce the risk of another event.

29
Statins:
The Magic Bullets

Statins are among our most powerful weapons for combating heart disease because they literally do help to unclog our arteries.

The word *statin* is derived from the Greek *statos* = 'fixed or stationary', implying 'to stop or halt'. It is a clever name for a family of drugs that reduces the body's production of cholesterol, lowering blood LDL levels as a result. Statins have become so well known that they featured on the cover of *Newsweek,* which published an eight-page summary of their remarkable benefits. These include:

- In clinical trials, 25–30 per cent lower risk of death, heart attack and stroke after five years of treatment when compared with inactive (placebo) treatment. This evidence for benefit in heart attack and stroke has been obtained in over 90,000 people and is perhaps the strongest for any treatment in medical practice.
- Possible lower risk of developing Alzheimer's disease (trials to confirm this are in progress).

- Possible lower risk of developing osteoporosis (trials in progress).
- Possible improvement in people with multiple sclerosis on the basis of animal experiments (trials in progress).
- Possible lower risk of progression of aortic valve thickening (trials in progress).
- Possible better outcome for those with heart failure (trials in progress).
- Possible lower risk of prostate cancer (trials not yet underway but in development stage).

Statins have shown the most rapid growth in use of any single drug and are the world's single top-selling pharmaceutical product, with doctors around the world writing more than 120 million prescriptions annually. The main reasons for this phenomenal growth are:

- The treatment of high cholesterol has been revolutionised by their use. Once difficult to control, cholesterol is now much more effectively treated with statins than ever before.
- In large clinical trials with over 90,000 subjects, statins have been proven to lower heart attack rates by 20–30 per cent.
- Clinical trials have also shown reduction in strokes, bypass surgery and angioplasty/stenting in those treated with statins compared with placebo (inactive tablets).
- Heart attack remains the single most frequent cause of death in developed nations—there are over 3.5 million deaths annually from heart attack worldwide, and numbers are increasing as Western populations age and Asian and third-world countries adopt Western lifestyles.
- Lower LDL levels are being recommended as more clinical trials show benefit from 'lower the better' LDL levels, particularly in those with previous heart attack or stroke; statins are the most effective drugs to lower LDL (by up to

55 per cent).

- Statins are more readily accepted by patients than older drugs to lower cholesterol because they are better tolerated.

Prophetic words

When I wrote my first book, *Cholesterol Control*, in 1986, I mentioned mevinolin (lovastatin) in the chapter on drug therapy for cholesterol:

'A drug that looks very promising at the present time is mevinolin, which reduces the production of cholesterol by the tissues, especially the liver. Mevinolin has been shown to reduce blood cholesterol/HDL ratios by about 45 per cent in people with high blood cholesterol levels of about 9 mmol/l, average levels falling to 6 mmol/l. Mevinolin increases the effectiveness of Questran, and when used together with Questran has been of particular value in the treatment of people with familial hypercholesterolaemia. Mevinolin has also recently been reported to be more effective when combined with either gemfibrozil, nicotinic acid, Colestid or probucol.'

Recent evidence suggests that many drugs lower blood cholesterol levels because they increase the number of LDL receptors in the tissues. This allows cholesterol to be removed from the blood and metabolised.

The era of drug treatment for high blood cholesterol levels has really just begun. Extensive research and development of new drugs for cholesterol control will very likely produce more effective and acceptable medications than are now available.'

These were prophetic words. In the late 1980s, the 'statin era' began. Since then, statins have truly revolutionised the practice of preventive medicine.

Chemical modification of lovastatin resulted in the development of two new semi-synthetic statins—simvastatin and pravastatin, which were marketed in the late 1980s. Then the synthetic statins were developed: fluvastatin, cerivastatin and atorvastatin.

Statins were very quickly found to have the following advantages over previously available drugs to lower cholesterol:

- Fewer side effects.
- More easily taken as a single tablet once a day.
- More pronounced lowering of LDL.

Statins also raised blood levels of HDL and lowered triglycerides (both beneficial effects).

Statin clinical trials

Clinical trials were soon begun to investigate whether statins worked in different people with a variety of background medical conditions, and if they also had advantages over existing drugs for lowering cholesterol. It was particularly important to show that statins lowered heart attack rates more effectively than previous medications.

These trials involved treating people with either a statin or an inactive tablet with an identical appearance to the active drug (a placebo). In this way, there was no bias in the study against either one or the other tablet, because both the patient and the investigator were blinded to the true identity of the tablets. The patient was also randomly allocated into either the placebo or the active-treatment arm of the study by computer, so that the study was *randomised* with regard to therapy. This also minimised bias and allowed a scientifically valid result to be obtained.

Let's look at results of the clinical trials with statins. These have involved over 90,000 subjects treated with either a statin or placebo for five years.

The results can be summarised simply as: every 1.0 reduction in LDL (for example dropping LDL from 6 to 5, or from 5 to 4) there was:

- 21 per cent lower rate of heart attacks, strokes, bypass operations and coronary angioplasties.
- 12 per cent lower death rate.

These results can be translated into numbers as follows:

- For those with previous heart attack, there were 48 less cardiovascular events over five years for every 1000 people treated.
- For those with no previous heart attack, there were 25 less major cardiovascular events over five years for every 1000 people treated.

The results also provided evidence for 'lower LDL is better'. There was a straight line relationship between vascular events and LDL reduction. For example, a 40 per cent lower event rate occurred in those with LDL reduction of 2.0, while a 10 per cent lower occurred in those with LDL reduction was 0.5.

The interpretation of these trials can be summarised simply.

1. For every 1.0 mmol/l lowering of LDL with a statin, there is about 20 per cent reduction over five years in heart attacks, strokes and revascularisation procedures (bypass surgery or balloon angioplasty) compared with placebo.
2. When LDL is lowered with statins, it has to be lowered as far as possible to achieve maximum benefits.

All of the trials also showed an increase in HDL levels as a result of statin treatment, which may account for a significant proportion (up to 30 per cent) of the overall benefits of statin therapy. This is because very small increases in HDL cholesterol are associated with large benefits in reducing cardiovascular risk.

The benefits of statin treatment occur equally in various subgroups, including diabetics and non–diabetics, men and women, young and old, and those with high and low cholesterol, normal and high blood pressure. Benefits are therefore independent of baseline characteristics and apply 'across the board' to everybody treated with statins.

What the experts say about statins

- 'An estimated one-third reduction in heart attacks, strokes and bypass surgery was the likely outcome from treatment

with a statin for five years.'
- 'Lowering cholesterol is beneficial in high-risk people even if cholesterol levels are as low as 3.5.'
- 'Safety and benefit is seen from lowering LDL down to 1.8.'
- 'It's never too late to treat high-risk people: benefits were seen even in those older than 75.'
- 'Statins should become first-line treatment to lower cholesterol in diabetics.'
- 'Benefits of lowering cholesterol were seen equally in men and women.'
- 'Current recommendations for treatment of high cholesterol are now outdated.'

The last point is very important and deserves more discussion. Clinical trials with statins have now shown benefit from lowering LDL as far as 1.8 in people who've had a heart attack. For this reason, recent expert panels have subsequently advised that lowering LDL to 1.8 may be appropriate (see Chapter 27).

Statin combination therapy

New drug combinations that include a statin have recently been introduced into the market, and more are on the way. These tablets will allow the benefits of different drugs to be conveniently combined in a single tablet, taken once a day, and include:
- pravastatin + aspirin (to prevent clotting)—available in US.
- atorvastatin + amlodipine (to lower blood pressure)— recently available in Australia.
- simvastatin + ezetimibe (to further lower LDL)— introduced in Australia in 2006.

Aspirin is an anti–clotting drug that lowers heart attack and stroke by 20–30 per cent (in those with previous cardiovascular disease). In combination with the statin pravastatin, we can expect a 40–55 per cent reduction in the risk of heart attack and stroke.

Amlodipine is a drug that lowers blood pressure and has a similar benefit to aspirin. In combination with the statin atorvastatin, we can expect a 50–70 per cent reduction in risk of heart attack and stroke.

Ezetimibe is a drug that lowers LDL by about 20 per cent (see Chapter 30 on new cholesterol-lowering drugs). In combination with the statin simvastatin, the risk of heart attack or stroke should be reduced by up to 70 per cent.

The polypill

The combination of various drugs with statins has been taken to another level by the suggestion that statins be combined with:

- An anti-clotting drug (low-dose aspirin)
- A drug to lower blood pressure (e.g. ACE inhibitor)
- A fluid tablet (also to lower blood pressure)
- Folic acid

Aspirin, ACE inhibitors and fluid tablets have all been shown to lower the risk of heart attacks, but evidence for folic acid is so far lacking. In theory, folic acid is beneficial because it lowers blood levels of the risk factor homocysteine.

The polypill has created lots of controversy among medical experts. On the one hand, its supporters recognise the advantages of a single daily tablet over multiple tablets, as single tablets are more likely to be taken and not left on the shelf. The additive benefits of each component of the polypill is likely to result in even lower heart attacks and strokes. Those who are more sceptical of the polypill say its benefits are overstated, and side effects may be increased by adding so many components together. The doses may also not be the right ones needed for a given individual. If we look at the way pharmaceutical products are heading, however, combination therapy is the way for the future. A clinical trial of the polypill is already underway in India, where it has been produced at a fraction of the cost in other countries.

Whether the polypill, or a modified version of it, ever comes to market is only speculation at the moment. My prediction is that it will, in a modified form and in varying doses, to allow some adjustment for individual prescription.

Other effects of statins

We have seen that statins lower the risk of both heart attacks and strokes. One reason for this is that statins lower LDL and triglycerides, and also raise HDL levels.

Other effects: these may be partly independent of their effects on blood cholesterol and triglycerides, and include:

- Improved blood flow to areas of the heart (and possibly other tissues such as the brain) that have insufficient blood supply.
- Reduced enlargement of heart muscle cells in response to high blood pressure.
- Reduced clotting tendency.
- Protection of LDL from oxidation.
- Protection of heart muscle from damage due to lack of blood supply.
- Improvement in heart failure.
- Lowering of blood pressure in combination with blood pressure-lowering drugs.
- Slowed progression of aortic valve thickening.
- Increased survival after heart transplantation.
- Changes in plaque composition and structure, consistent with increased plaque stability.

Statins stabilise plaques

The end result of statin treatment is to transform dangerous plaques into less dangerous ones that are less likely to rupture. Cooling off plaques is one way to describe this process, as though a volcano about to erupt were cooled down and rendered quiescent.

Another way is to think in terms of plaque solidity. A vulnerable plaque is soft and jelly-like, and prone to deformation in response to physical injury (as occurs with each heartbeat, when the arterial wall flexes back and forth). A less vulnerable plaque is firmer, and undergoes less deformation with injury. The plaque has been 'solidified'. An analogy is cement-making, when solidification is made possible by adding lime to the mixture of sand, water and cement. Statins, like lime, act as 'solidifying' agents, making plaques less vulnerable to rupture.

Taking care with statins

However, those on statins need to be more aware of any unusual muscle or joint aches and pains. We have seen that the incidence of reported muscle and joint side effects in statin trials was similar in placebo-treated and statin-treated groups. These results are reassuring. Similar results apply to many other adverse events with statins, whether related to the stomach, intestines, nerves, skin, or other organs.

Muscle aches and pains are very common. Statins are commonly prescribed. So add the two together and there will be a lot of people complaining of muscle aches and pains while on statin therapy. In the majority of cases, statins are not responsible for the aches and pains. In some, they may be aggravating 'normal' symptoms. In a very few, significant muscle damage may occur. It is important to rule out low thyroid activity in a person suffering from aches and pains while being treated with a statin.

Side effects must be placed in context of the reason for prescribing statins in the first place. Statins are life-saving drugs. They significantly reduce rates of heart attacks, strokes and death in the short term, and are likely to have even greater benefits in the longer term. Statins should not be stopped unless there is clear evidence of significant adverse effects.

There is, however, a very uncommon and serious condition, that can occur in about one per million statin prescriptions, called *rhabdomyolysis* (from the Greek *rhabdos* = rod, *mus* = muscle and *luo* = dissolve). This condition is also known as 'muscle melt-down', and is most frequently seen in runners with heat exhaustion. It can also occur after surgery, extensive trauma and with kidney failure. It causes weakness, stiffness, aching and pain in the muscles to the extent that it may be difficult to get out of a chair, raise the arms above the head or walk quickly. The muscles may also be tender to pressure.

Any minor degree of damage to muscles (such as a punch on the arm, or even vigorous exercise) allows enzymes within the muscle cells to leak out into the blood. One of these enzymes, creatine kinase (CK), can be measured and its level indicates the degree of muscle damage. Normal levels are less than 160–200 (this varies in different laboratories), and minor damage can result in levels 2–3 times higher than the upper range of normal.

With muscle melt-down, CK levels are usually more than 40 times higher than normal (over 6000), indicating extensive muscle damage. Risk factors for muscle melt-down with statin treatment include:

- Use of high-dose statins in thin elderly people.
- Combination therapy of statin and a cholesterol-lowering drug called gemfibrozil.
- Other conditions increasing the likelihood of muscle cell damage, including major surgery, severe acute infection and extensive trauma as in road accidents.
- Impaired kidney and liver function.
- Low thyroid activity. This is a particularly important predisposing factor because of its frequency among elderly women. It may cause muscle aches and pains on statin treatment, as well as lethargy, lack of energy, sensitivity to cold, dry skin, hair thinning and hair loss, constipation, weight gain and swelling of ankles.
- Low blood sodium.
- Uncontrolled seizures.
- Low body temperature.
- Low oxygen levels.
- Drugs of abuse (alcohol, cocaine, ecstasy, lysergide, amphetamines).

Most clinicians recommend using the lowest statin dose necessary to achieve satisfactory LDL levels in order to minimise side effects and to prevent statin blood levels from becoming too high. This is especially important in those with low body weight, such as thin elderly people, who may also have impaired liver and kidney function that can inhibit the body's metabolism of statins.

If you are taking a statin you should report any unusual muscle aches and pains to your doctor as soon as possible. Don't adopt a wait-and-see policy. Your doctor will have explained this to you when you were given the first prescription for the statin. Don't hesitate. If you have a sudden onset of muscle aches, see your doctor. It may or may not be caused by the drug, but both you and your doctor will want to check it out.

SUMMARY

- The results of statin therapy have been more than gratifying—some would say miraculous. A significantly lower rate of heart attacks and strokes has been achieved without an increase in any other serious condition, particularly cancer. Statins as a group are also well-tolerated and convenient to take in a once-daily dose.
- Statins have become drugs of first choice for cholesterol control throughout the world, and account for a significant proportion of the health expenditure of many countries.
- There is no specific treatment for statin muscle aches and pains other than stopping the statin, then trying a lower statin dose, and if this is not successful, a different statin.
- The mechanism of muscle damage has yet to be defined.
- Inform your doctor if you experience any unusual muscle aches or pains, muscle weakness or tenderness.
- Check with your pharmacist if other drugs you are taking may be interacting with the statin.
- If in doubt, stop taking the statin and see your doctor at the earliest opportunity.

30
The Latest
and Greatest
Medications

In Chapter 1, we discussed how the body forms collateral circulation routes (nature's bypasses) at sites of severe clogging of the arteries. In this way, blood flow beyond the site of clogging can be maintained. Some drugs are currently being developed that can create a collateral circulation when injected into clogged arteries, but routine use is some years away.

The development of statins has made an enormous difference to medical practice over the last 15 years. Statin treatment can unclog the arteries and reduce the risk of heart attack and stroke. But it's important to realise that those taking statins can still suffer heart attacks, albeit at a significantly lower rate. Treatment with current drugs is a powerful weapon. It is not, however, the end of the war. The search therefore continues for new medications to control clogging of the arteries that will be even more effective in controlling cholesterol, reducing heart attacks and strokes, and saving lives.

Some of the new medications include:

- Bile acid binding agents
- Cholesterol absorption inhibitors
- ACAT inhibitors
- CETP blockers
- Plant stanols and sterols
- PPAR alpha stimulants
- Recombinant apo A-1 Milano

Bile acid binding agents

The latest of this class of medications is colesavelam, which like cholestyramine (Questran) and colestipol (Colestid), binds to bile acids in the intestine and prevents their absorption into the blood. As a result, the liver removes more LDL from the blood by increasing the activity of its LDL receptors. Lower blood LDL levels are the end result.

Cholestyramine and colestipol are powders that need to be mixed with fluid. They are relatively unpalatable and difficult to take in the long term. Colesavelam is in tablet form, the usual dose being six tablets daily (3.8g). At this dose, LDL levels are reduced by 15 per cent on average.

Colesavelam, like the other bile acid binders, is very effective in combination with statins. For example, LDL can be lowered by about 40 per cent by colesavelam taken with 10 mg/day of simvastatin.

Colesavelam is also tolerated better than the older powders, and has less tendency to raise triglyceride levels.

Cholesterol absorption inhibitors

The first of these, ezetimibe (Ezetrol), reduces the absorption of cholesterol from the intestine, thereby lowering blood LDL levels by about 18 per cent at a daily dose of 10 mg. Ezetimibe accumulates just under the surface layer of the cells lining the small intestine, from where it is absorbed into the body and excreted into the bile by the liver. It is recycled from the liver to the intestines via the bile just like cholesterol and bile acids.

Ezetimibe prevents cholesterol absorption by binding to a specific transport protein (NCP1L1) that is responsible for absorption of both cholesterol and plant sterols. For this reason it is also used to treat people with a rare genetic disorder, beta-sitosterolaemia, in which excessive absorption of a plant sterol called beta-sitosterol leads to its accumulation in the blood and clogging of the arteries.

Ezetimibe appears to be safe when taken with statins and all other types of cholesterol-lowering medications.

Lowering LDL by 18–20 per cent is equivalent to three doublings or dose titrations of a given statin, so that ezetimibe will probably be most useful when combined with a low-dose statin. In this way any side effects associated with higher statin doses may be avoided, while providing greater cholesterol control. Such a principle is already established for blood pressure control, in which small doses of two or more medications are often used instead of higher doses of one medication.

The combination medication Vytorin (ezetimibe + simvastatin in a single tablet) has recently been introduced in Australia, with simvastatin in doses of either 40 mg or 80 mg. The PBS in Australia has recently approved combining ezetimibe with lower statin doses in people who cannot tolerate 40-80 mg of statin daily.

ACAT inhibitors

ACAT is an enzyme that acts to add a fatty acid molecule to choles-terol, thereby forming a cholesterol ester. Cholesterol esters are more fat-soluble than cholesterol, and are stored in cells within fat droplets.

Inhibiting the ACAT enzyme is of theoretical benefit by inhibiting the formation of cholesterol ester-rich cells in the early phases of clogging of the arteries.

The ACAT inhibitor pactimibe has been shown to reduce clogging of the arteries in experimental animals. A recent controlled clinical trial, however, showed that pactimibe did not reduce the rate of heart attacks, so that further marketing of this particular ACAT inhibitor may not occur.

Plant stanols and sterols

Plants do not contain cholesterol. Instead, they contain plant *stanols* (campestanol and sitostanol) and *sterols* (campesterol and sitosterol), which are closely related to cholesterol in chemical structure.

Humans do not absorb dietary plant stanols. Plant sterols are absorbed like cholesterol by the NCP1L1 protein previously discussed in relation to ezetimibe. Both plant sterols and stanols compete with dietary cholesterol for absorption, lowering the absorption of cholesterol and lowering blood LDL levels by up-regulation of the liver's LDL receptors.

Plant sterols occur in small quantities in plants but have been processed by esterification (addition of a fatty acid) to enable them to be concentrated in enriched margarines, which contain about 2 g of plant sterol esters per 20 g of margarine. Between 2–3 g daily of plant sterols are necessary to lower LDL levels by 10–15 per cent, so a relatively large amount of margarine needs to be consumed (20–30 g daily is the amount in 2–3 tablespoons).

Plant sterols have been shown to lower LDL by an additional 10 per cent when taken in conjunction with a cholesterol-lowering diet or statins. Plant sterol supplements may also reduce the absorption of fat soluble beta-carotenes from yellow and orange fruits and vegetables, so more of these should be eaten when taking plant sterols.

CETP inhibitors

Cholesterol ester transfer protein (CETP) is a key enzyme in the pathway of HDL metabolism. It transfers cholesterol from HDL to other lipoproteins (VLDL and LDL) in exchange for triglycerides.

Inhibition of CETP therefore increases the amount of cholesterol in HDL—a theoretically beneficial change. Two CETP inhibitors have been developed so far: JTT-705 and torcetrapib. Torcetrapib increases

HDL by 16–91 per cent in doses from 10–120 mg daily, and also reduces LDL by 21–42 per cent. These effects were expected to be beneficial, but a recent trial of torcetrapib was stopped prematurely because of increased heart attacks. As a result, the drug was withdrawn from further development.

PPAR alpha stimulants

PPAR stands for *peroxisome proliferator activated receptor* and refers to a family of proteins that control the metabolism of fatty acids, glucose, cholesterol and triglycerides, and the development of fat (adipose) and other tissues.

Both fibrates and statins activate PPAR α, which alters the activity of 80–100 genes, switching some on and others off. The end result of this is:

- Increasing the production of HDL proteins.
- Increasing the breakdown of triglycerides in lipoproteins.
- Increasing the production of a protein (ABCA-1) that transports cholesterol out of cells into the blood, where it is picked up HDL.
- Increasing the production of a receptor that removes cholesterol from tissues.

All these effects raise blood HDL levels, lower tissue cholesterol levels and should inhibit clogging of the arteries. PPAR α activation also switches on genes that have anti-inflammatory and anti-clotting actions, and others that can prevent damage to the lining of the blood vessels.

The cholesterol-lowering fibrates act directly to stimulate PPAR α, while statins are thought to act indirectly via alteration of a signalling pathway.

Several different PPARα molecules are in development, but it will be several years before they are ready for marketing.

HDL-like proteins

The HDL-like proteins are similar in structure to apoA-1, the major protein of HDL. The first of these, apo A-1 Milano, is a fascinating example of Pasteur's dictum, 'Chance favours the prepared mind.'

Limone sul Garda, a small village near Milan, was found to have many long-lived inhabitants distinguished not only by their birth certificates but also by the fact that their levels of HDL were low. This was a paradoxical situation, for low HDL levels should have led to premature heart attack and reduced life expectancy.

It was suggested that low HDL levels in the Limonese resulted from accelerated removal of HDL cholesterol by the liver. In this way, cholesterol build-up and clogging of the arteries was prevented. An Italian research team discovered a change in the protein structure of apo A-1 due to a genetic variant. The new apo A-1 was called apo A-1 Milano.

The method for isolating the protein was patented and developed. In November 2003, a small study showed that several weekly injections of a new compound based on apo A-1 Milano (code-named ETC-216) reduced the size of coronary artery plaques by about 4 per cent. Studies on the use of ETC-216 are underway, and the results are awaited with great interest as the medication may prove to be a novel way to slow down clogging of the arteries.

SUMMARY

- In this modern age we are accustomed to the 'magic bullet' approach to solving medical problems through taking a pill. The prime example of this is the remarkable success of the cholesterol-lowering drugs called statins.
- Statins have revolutionised medical practice and been shown to unclog the arteries and reduce rates of heart attack and stroke. The health impact of statins has been likened to that of antibiotics. Little wonder, therefore, that the search continues for more effective medications to lower cholesterol, LDL and triglycerides.
- The search to find medications to raise HDL has taken a battering from the withdrawal of torcetrapib, but other candidates are being hotly pursued. There seems little doubt that more 'magic bullets' will be found, hopefully with even more dramatic benefits than antibiotics and statins.

31
Lowering Triglyceride Levels with Drugs

Triglycerides are the 'forgotten fats', and are often neglected in programs to control risk factors.

We have discussed what triglycerides are—their chemical composition and their function (see Chapter 8). To recap, triglycerides are essential components of the body that have two basic functions:

- To insulate the body against heat loss (the layer of fat beneath the skin is composed mainly of triglycerides).
- To provide energy for metabolism (the body's fat stores under the skin, inside the abdomen and within cells of muscles and the liver are composed of triglycerides).

Here we focuses on how triglycerides contribute to clogging of the arteries and how drugs are used to control their levels in the blood.

Humans have evolved a complex series of chemical reactions by which dietary energy (in the form of fat, carbohydrate and protein) can be converted to storage fat, and vice-versa.

During periods of fasting or famine, triglycerides in storage fat can be broken down to fatty acids and glycerol. Fatty acids can then be oxidised to carbon dioxide and water, releasing heat and energy.

During periods of feasting, dietary fats are stored in subcutaneous and visceral fat.

Triglycerides are predominantly transported in the blood within the triglyceride-rich particles called chylomicrons and very low-density lipoproteins (VLDL).

The metabolism of triglycerides is intimately linked to that of cholesterol, LDL and HDL. Altered triglyceride metabolism can have significant effects on LDL and HDL levels, and therefore increase the risk of cardiovascular disease.

One key concept is the 'seesaw' relationship between levels of triglycerides and HDL. When TG levels are low, HDL levels tend to be high, and vice-versa.

Because of the dynamic relationship between LDL, HDL and triglycerides, it is not physiologically valid to consider each of these blood fats as a separate entity. This is done, nevertheless, when blood fats are measured and correlated with cardiovascular events in clinical trials.

What is the evidence linking triglycerides with vascular disease?

1. Population studies have shown increased blood triglycerides to be associated with increased cardiovascular risk.

An overall analysis of several studies which followed over 45,000 men and 10,000 women for up to 11 years showed for every 1.0 increase in blood triglycerides, heart attack rates increased by 14 per cent in men and 37 per cent in women. The analysis adjusted for levels of other risk factors, including HDL.

In some individual studies, however, the relationship disappeared when levels of HDL were taken into account (suggesting that triglycerides may be only a marker for low HDL, at least in statistical terms).

For this reason, triglycerides have long been considered less important risk factors than HDL—triglycerides have been the 'forgotten fats'.

One of the reasons for lack of correlation between triglycerides and vascular disease in some population studies is that there is quite a wide variation in triglyceride levels within any individual on a day-to-day basis. This lowers the power of a statistical test to show a relationship between triglycerides and risk.

2. High blood triglycerides are associated with other cardiovascular risk factors.

These include small, dense LDL, a protein called apoB, and various clotting factors.

Small dense LDL

When triglyceride levels are higher than about 1.7, there is a shift in the size and structure of LDL molecules in the blood. LDL particles become smaller and more dense, and more prone to accumulate in the vessel walls and promote atherosclerosis (hardening of the arteries) compared with normal large, less dense LDL.

ApoB

Each VLDL and LDL particle has one molecule of apoB. VLDL are metabolised to LDL, and the apoB of LDL is recognised by the LDL receptor on the surface of liver cells.

Blood levels of apoB therefore reflect levels of both VLDL and LDL, and reflect the rate of transport of cholesterol into the arterial wall and risk of hardening of the arteries.

Clotting factors

Where blood triglycerides are high, clotting factors are increased, and may increase the tendency for thrombosis, leading to a heightened risk of heart attack.

Genetic disorders of triglyceride metabolism can be associated with premature cardiovascular diseases.

These disorders are characterised by increased blood triglycerides, as well as increased levels of cholesterol. They are discussed in Chapter 11, and include familial hypertriglyceridaemia and familial combined hyperlipidaemia. The origin and metabolism of blood triglycerides is discussed in Chapter 8.

Drugs for controlling triglycerides

Many of the drugs that lower triglycerides also lower cholesterol, because they are transported together in lipoproteins and are linked metabolically.

Statins

These drugs are generally more powerful at lowering cholesterol than triglycerides, other than in high doses, when statins may be very effective agents for lowering triglycerides. Statins lower triglycerides by reducing the liver's secretion of VLDL.

Statins have little effect on triglycerides below about 2.0. Above this, the effect of statins depends on the dose of statin and the level of triglycerides. Higher doses are more effective. The higher the triglyceride level, the greater the reduction.

In people with mildly elevated triglycerides, a reduction of 15–20 per cent is usually seen with average dose statin treatment.

Statins that are more powerful in lowering LDL are also more powerful in lowering triglycerides.

Statins have been shown in many clinical trials to lower heart attack rates as well as rates of stroke and bypass surgery.

Fibrates

Fibrates are derivatives of *fibric acid*, and members of this family include clofibrate, bezafibrate, ciprofibrate, gemfibrozil and fenofibrate. In Australia, only gemfibrozil (Lopid, Jezil) and fenofibrate (Lipidil) are available, after clofibrate was withdrawn from the market in the early 1990s after sales dropped with the availability of gemfibrozil.

Fibrates have multiple actions on fat metabolism and are especially effective in lowering triglycerides, while at the same time raising protective HDL levels. They are less effective on LDL levels, which may actually increase in some people.

Fibrates can lower triglycerides by more than 50 per cent (especially when they are very high). Even greater lowering of triglycerides occurs when fibrates are taken in conjunction with either statins or fish oils.

There are several published trials showing lower rates of cardiovascular disease with fibrate treatment. Benefits observed were probably the result of several mechanisms, including lowering triglycerides, raising HDL, and reducing the tendency of blood clotting or thrombosis.

A recent study of fenofibrate also showed:

- Less damage to the kidneys, as measured by albumin excretion in the urine (*microalbuminuria*).
- Less damage to the arteries of the eye, as measured by the number of laser treatments required (30 per cent lower than the placebo group).

Summary of fibrate trials

Almost 40,000 people have now been randomised to treatment with either a placebo or a fibrate (in some trials to nicotinic acid as well, or nicotinic acid in combination with a fibrate).

The heart attack rate was lowered on average by 29 per cent with fibrate treatment (with a wide range from 0 to 68 per cent).

The most conspicuous change in blood fats with fibrate treatment was lowering of blood triglycerides (28 per cent on average). This was a much greater change than cholesterol (8.5 per cent lower), LDL (7 per cent lower) and HDL (8 per cent higher).

The baseline blood cholesterol levels varied widely from 4.5–7.5, but the patient groups were selected to have baseline triglycerides below 4.5 (to allow calculation of LDL levels, which is not possible when TG are above 4.5).

Most of the subjects were men, and most were middle-aged (there were no people over the age of 75).

In a strictly scientific sense, the restrictions in inclusion criteria do not allow extrapolation of the results of the fibrate trials to other populations with different characteristics, but other than for the FIELD Study, there is good general agreement between the trials in terms of overall benefits in lowering heart attack rates, whether in people with or without previous heart attack.

Fish oils

We discussed fish oils in Chapter 14. They are very effective in lowering triglycerides, and can be taken with statins, fibrates and other cholesterol lowering medications. Fish oils have unusual biological properties that include:
- Lowering the liver's production of triglycerides
- Anti-inflammatory effects
- Suppression of immune functions
- Anti-clotting effects
- Suppressing heart rhythm disturbances
- Lowering blood pressure
- Antioxidant effects

Because of these effects, fish oils have been used successfully to treat a variety of joint disorders.

Nicotinic acid

Nicotinic acid is useful for controlling triglycerides if tolerated). Mega-doses (1–3g daily) are often required and can lower triglycerides by up to 50 per cent as well as lowering cholesterol and LDL (by 15–30 per cent). HDL may also increase by up to 30 per cent.

SUMMARY

- Triglycerides are a critical link between LDL, HDL and risk of cardiovascular disease.
- Raised triglycerides may be the first sign of diabetes (see Chapter 21).
- Raised triglycerides increase cardiovascular risk by several mechanisms, including an increased tendency to blood clotting.
- Controlled clinical trials of drugs to lower triglycerides show beneficial effects in reducing cardiovascular risk.
- Lifestyle is also important to control triglycerides: one of these is the SAFE program (see Chapter 24).

32
Tablets Only Work if You Take Them

Less than a medical generation ago, patients were not happy unless they left the doctor's surgery with a fistful of prescriptions. We were in the middle of the 'super pill' era, when there was a magic bullet for everything from ingrown toenails to weight loss.

This era followed the ubiquitous 'era of the bottle'. A few generations before me, doctors used to dispense their cures in small and mysterious brown glass bottles with corks. Patients used to literally come in to see the doctor and say, 'Doctor, I have a pain—can you give me a bottle for it?'

The 'bottle era', of course, was the era of faith. Some wise old family physicians used to brew up a bottle of what was essentially sugar syrup and a few herbs to make it taste bitter. Patients would happily go off and feel better for taking something they believed was doing them good. Was the clinician acting ethically? Those were the days of treating through personal experience rather than on the basis of large scientific studies. The doctor had no other 'cure', and did the best he could by literally giving hope in a bottle.

Today, of course, the patient has the right to know what is going on. We discuss the medication in detail, hand out pamphlets, other reading matter and even sometimes CDs. Often the patient knows almost as much about the medication as the doctor. (Or at least, many think they do!)

Not surprisingly, this steep rise in knowledge has led to lowered rates of compliance. According to the dictionary, compliance means 'action in response to a request or command'. A compliant person is one who does what he or she is asked to do (from the Latin *complere*, to complete).

Nowadays it's the old story of a little knowledge sometimes being a dangerous thing. All medications, for example, can have side effects, but if a patient reads up on all the side effects too thoroughly, he or she may begin to imagine having them. It's a bit like the medical student who always thinks he or she has the disease which is being studied. I had that experience myself, and so did many of my friends.

So compliance is all about not only working out the correct medical regimen for a patient, but also making it as comfortable, rewarding and as positive an experience as possible, so the patient will stick to the medication. Compliance is a major issue for the clinician as well as the patient.

Doctors are faced every day with patients who say they have read or seen on TV extravagant claims for health benefits of a variety of 'miracle' medications, often promoted by those who have no knowledge of science and are happy to be paid handsomely for presenting to the public. Some of these so-called medications are not well tested by international scientific study standards.

We also have to consider the evidence-based medicine that we have discussed, which means only treat with a tablet if there is scientific evidence that it works.

Doctors are happy to dispense their medications, give advice on what they are for, what side effects may occur, and arrange to see the patient again after a certain number of weeks to check how they are getting on.

Many patients are happy to get a prescription, then leave it in the car or in the kitchen drawer, and think about whether they really need it before taking it to the pharmacist. Some of these patients never get to the pharmacy at all. Others do eventually go, then read the package insert, and say to themselves, 'I wouldn't take this in a thousand years!'

The ideal patient, of course, *is* compliant. He or she:

- First and foremost, understands why the tablets are necessary.
- Obeys instructions to the letter.
- Has been given a full explanation by the doctor.
- Receives the same information from the chemist, thereby reinforcing the doctor's message.
- Reads the package insert without worrying that every possible side effect mentioned might or probably will occur.
- Is willing to ask questions right at the beginning and to ring for advice if there is any area of uncertainty, having been invited to do so by the doctor.
- Understands fully what the tablets are designed to do, how they should be taken, possible interactions with other medications, and how long they need to be taken for.

There are two real issues of compliance:

The Plus-Factor

Firstly, the patient needs positive input, i.e. a sense of purpose and a feeling of empowerment because by taking the appropriate medication, he or she is taking a positive step towards gaining and maintaining continuing good cardiac health. This is the Plus-Factor.

The Minus-Factor

Secondly, there is the Minus-Factor. This is the 'lack of negative input'. By taking this medication, the patient is not in some way diminishing his or her lifestyle or increasing the chance of side effects.

It is vital for the clinician and the patient to take seriously and to address successfully both of these issues.

With positive input, the patient needs continuous reassurance that the tablets are the right ones for his or her needs and they are doing the job. This means a reasonable amount of clinical supervision. These days, there are issues of so-called over-servicing which conscientious clinicians are at pains to avoid. But doctors must be very careful not to under-service patients, who need to be encouraged and reassured. They can tell their patients to call at a certain time if necessary. This gives them a sense of continuous contact, even when they do not—as most don't—regularly take advantage of it.

Patients need to have regular blood tests to see their improving results. It is like anything else in life, from golf to learning a language: if you see improvement, even with the occasional setback, you will be far more likely to continue with the project.

In lowering LDL, the patient and the clinician are a team working together for a common purpose or goal. If both make sure they understand this, you are on the road to good compliance. 'We are going to do this—together' is the best way, in my experience, of introducing the need for medication. This is ideally followed by a series of small victories which you achieve together and on which you can congratulate each other. This sounds simple, but it really does work.

The negative factor is, in some ways—or more correctly, in some people—more difficult to control. Basically, it means making sure there are no unpleasant, lifestyle-altering side effects.

The doctor will routinely ask each patient at follow-up visits if there are any problems with taking medication, and the patient must volunteer symptoms about which he or she is concerned.

Without being neurotic, a person on medication must look out for any untoward or unusual symptoms which may be a result of the medication *and report them*.

Not only are we looking for the obvious medical complications, but also the lifestyle-altering issues which may finally make the patient throw up his or her hands in despair and say: 'I'm not going to put up with this' and instead of coming in to discuss it with the doctor, flushes the tablets down the lavatory. Then, feeling a bit embarrassed by doing so, never goes near the prescribing practitioner again.

One only has to look at organisations such as Weight Watchers, to see how a good game-plan plus continuous follow-up with positive reinforcement for goal achievement is the ideal manner for compliance. I often think a sort of Cholesterol Club, where patients can get together with a group leader to discuss their issues and to give encouragement to and learn from each other would be a positive initiative.

The science of compliance

My colleague, Professor Leon Simons and his wife Judy, have carried out some well-conceived and important studies on compliance. They first looked at prescriptions in Sydney for cholesterol-lowering drugs over a 12-month period in 1994–95. After one month, 15 per cent of prescriptions had been discontinued. A further 30 per cent was discontinued after three months, and a further 15 per cent discontinued over the next eight months. Only 40 per cent of prescriptions were taken after 12 months!

The main reasons for discontinuation were:
- Lack of conviction that the tablets were really necessary (lack of the Plus-Factor) in 32 per cent of cases.
- Lack of cholesterol-lowering in 32 per cent.
- Side effects (the Minus-Factor) in only 7 per cent.

Patients with cardiovascular disease or symptoms took their medications more regularly than patients without symptoms.

The Simons' next study in 1999 was to look at discontinuation rates for cholesterol-lowering medications Australia-wide using Medicare data. After six months, 30 per cent of prescriptions were discontinued. Over 90 per cent were for statins.

As you can imagine, these results created quite a stir in medical and administrative circles, and pointed out that more attention needed to be paid to compliance and surrounding issues.

Other studies in the US showed that giving cholesterol–lowering tablets in hospital during admission for coronary disease (whether for heart attack, unstable angina, bypass surgery or coronary angiography) led to a better compliance rate than delaying treatment until recovery. This policy of 'strike while the iron is hot' is now accepted in many centres worldwide. Here is a checklist to help improve compliance:

The Plus–Factor
- Why are the tablets being taken?
- What are the benefits in the short and long term?
- Will I live longer?
- Will I feel better?

In terms of cardiovascular disease, LDL–lowering medications have been shown to reduce the rate of heart attacks, sudden deaths, strokes (cerebral infarction and transient ischaemic attacks), bypass surgery, hospital admissions, and disability from stroke, angina and heart failure. The quality of life is improved because of these benefits. Overall health–care costs in the longer term are also reduced. Longevity is likely to be improved, especially when treating younger patients at higher risk.

LDL–lowering medications have also been shown to reduce the rate of progression and induce regression of atherosclerotic plaques.

For many years I have performed repeat carotid artery ultrasound tests on patients taking cholesterol-lowering medications. There is no better aid to compliance than demonstrating improvement in plaque size, or even regression of plaques, which occurs quite often after several years of consistent treatment.

Simply measuring blood fat levels and showing improvement with treatment is also a very effective way to improve compliance—if the results are good, there is a reason to take the medication. Remember: for every 1 per cent lowering of LDL cholesterol there is a 1–2 per cent reduction in heart attack, stroke, and bypass surgery over about five years of treatment.

For every 1 per cent increase in HDL cholesterol there is also a 1–2 per cent reduction in heart attack rates over the same period.

Longer periods of treatment are likely to result in further reduction in cardiovascular disease.

The Minus-Factor

- Will the medications affect my lifestyle? (For example, sexual function, libido, energy levels, sleep, alertness, appetite, irritability, emotional state, exercise capacity)
- Will the medications cause other side effects?

Of course, there is a long list of potential side effects with any medication, but the most common ones are listed in the package inserts. Many side effects are actually coincidental and have nothing to do with the medication.

One way to investigate this possibility (other than taking placebo tablets) is the withdraw-and-rechallenge test. This means stopping the medication for a defined period, keeping a close eye on whatever the side effect may be (or, in the case of problems with blood test results, repeating the blood test), and then going back on the medication to see what happens. This is a semi-scientific method but will often help to decide whether or not to keep taking the tablet, to change the dose, or to change to alternative medication.

An important point to remember is that the rates of side effects of cholesterol-lowering medications in clinical trials is similar for placebo and active-treatment groups. Minor side effects such as abdominal fullness and indigestion are relatively common (up to 10 per cent) but serious ones quite rare.

The Support-Factor

- Bring along a partner, spouse or close friend or relative to the consultation to have a 'second pair of ears'.
- Attend a Cholesterol Club support group where people can openly discuss problems and chat informally with clinicians.
- Check out information on the web (realising that this may be anecdotal and unsupported by scientific evidence).

Tricks of the trade

- Some people prefer to take their medications at a certain time each day. That's fine; usually this will not greatly alter the effectiveness of medications.
- Dosettes (little boxes divided into the days of the week, and morning and evening doses) often help those on multiple medications to remember to take them.
- Calendar packs marked from 1–28 days and the days of the week are now routinely available (having been initiated by manufacturers of 'the pill').
- Counting tablets left at the end of the month will determine how many were actually not taken. You can do better next month!
- Pharmacists are very willing to help discuss issues of side effects and interactions between different drugs—this is also their area of expertise.

SUMMARY

- Compliance (or more usually, lack of compliance) is a major problem.
- A tablet left on the shelf won't do anyone any good.
- There are ways to improve regular tablet-taking.

33
Surgery and Mechanical Unclogging

Many people experience silent clogging of the arteries over many years, until they develop symptoms related to lack of blood supply to the brain, heart, legs or other areas. When investigated, their arteries are found to be so badly clogged that urgent restoration of blood supply is necessary to prevent serious complications such as heart attack or stroke, as well as to control symptoms. In this chapter, we'll learn about the kinds of procedure—surgical and mechanical devices—used to deal with the problem of severely-clogged arteries.

Endarterectomy

Plaque can be removed under direct vision during a surgical procedure called *endarterectomy*. This is simply reaming out the hard plaque inside an artery after it has been opened by a small incision (after clamping both sides to prevent blood loss). Endarterectomy is most often used to unclog the carotid arteries when they are causing symptoms (we have discussed transient ischaemic attacks in Chapter 1). The patient will then take aspirin permanently after the procedure, and it is essential that they control the risk factors associated with clogging (see Chapter 5).

Endarterectomy of the coronary arteries was eventually disbanded because of poor results—the arteries clogged up again, probably because coronary arteries are too small to allow sufficient blood flow to prevent clotting after the procedure.

Athrectomy

Plaque can also be drilled away during a coronary angiogram using a tiny rotating device on the end of a catheter that has been inserted into the cavity of the artery. This procedure is called *athrectomy*. Several kinds of devices are available: one is an abrasive burr that grinds the plaque into small dust-like particles; another is a rotating blade that shaves the plaque and collects it in the tip of the catheter.

Athrectomy is mainly used to unclog calcified plaques that are blocking the artery, and is usually followed by angioplasty and stenting as we'll now discuss.

Angioplasty

Angioplasty is one of the miracles of modern medicine. It involves inserting into a narrowed coronary artery a catheter that has a tiny deflated balloon at the tip. The balloon is advanced across the site of narrowing and inflated under several atmospheres of pressure. The surrounding atherosclerotic plaque is compressed and blood flow restored (see Figures 33.1).

Angioplasty is one of the most frequently performed procedures, partly because clogging of the arteries is so common in our community, and partly because the results—relief of chest pain—have been so impressive.

Due to an increasingly steep learning curve over the past few years, cardiologists have become highly skilled in the procedure. There have also been remarkable improvements in technology, with a wide variety of catheters and balloons now used. These days, angioplasty is performed routinely in many centres throughout the world. It takes less than half an hour, several areas of clogging can be angioplastied during one procedure, and anginal chest pain is relieved.

Figure 33.1. Balloon angioplasty.

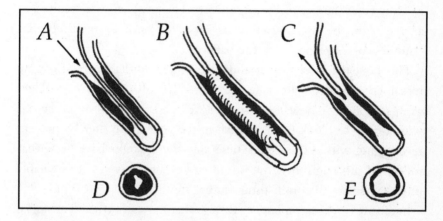

A: *catheter crosses the obstruction.*
B: *balloon is inflated, compressing the underlying plaque.*
C: *the catheter is withdrawn.*
D: *cross-section of artery before angioplasty.*
E: *Cross section of artery after angioplasty.*

Because of a 20–30 per cent rate of restenosis at the site of balloon angioplasty (where the artery returns to its narrowed state) after about six months, new procedures have been developed. The most successful is the use of wire baskets called stents, which are placed immediately after balloon angioplasty at the site. The stent not only keeps the artery open in a mechanical sense, but new stents are also available which are impregnated with a drug to prevent re-blockage by inhibiting the growth of cells in the underlying plaque. These 'eluting' stents are very expensive but have a very low rate of re-blockage.

Stenting

The main problem with early angioplasties was that up to 30 per cent of patients started to complain of chest pain within six months of the procedure. Repeat coronary angiograms showed that the artery had re-clogged at the site of the angioplasty. This problem was resolved to a large degree by inserting a wire basket called a *stent* immediately after compression of plaque with the balloon.

This kept the artery open and gave better results, but re-clogging remained a problem for a few patients. To solve this new problem of *in-stent stenosis*, new stents were developed that were impregnated with a drug to block tissue growth in the artery, and thereby prevent re-clogging within the stent. These *drug-eluting* stents have been very successful, although their use is limited because they are considerably more expensive than non–drug-eluting stents.

In recent years, angioplasty of the coronary arteries with stenting has become a more frequent procedure than bypass surgery.

Clot-busters

These are drugs that dissolve thrombi (clots) on the surface of ruptured plaques. The thrombi are responsible for blocking off blood supply to the tissue, so dissolving them will open up the vessel and restore flow. The medical term for clot-busting drugs is 'fibrinolytics'.

Clot-busters need to be given during the first few hours after the onset of symptoms to be effective. Recent trials have shown that immediate angioplasty and stenting of a blocked coronary artery gives better results than clot-busting drugs, so this is used in larger cities with angiography suites and experienced staff available.

Coronary bypass

Coronary bypass surgery involves creating another channel for blood to flow around the site of a severe obstruction by joining a small length of vein between the aorta and the coronary artery beyond its site of obstruction (see Figure 33.2). Alternatively, an artery can be used (usually the internal mammary artery, which runs down the inside of the sternum). After bypass, blood can now flow directly from the aorta to the coronary artery beyond the blockage.

Figure 33.2. Coronary bypass

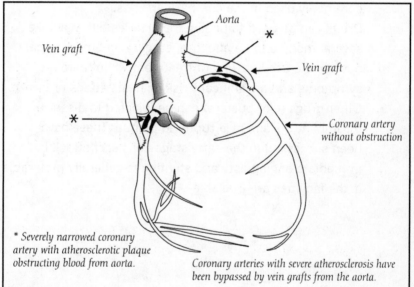

Aorta

Vein graft

*

Vein graft

*

Coronary artery
without obstruction

* Severely narrowed coronary
artery with atherosclerotic plaque
obstructing blood from aorta.

Coronary arteries with severe atherosclerosis have
been bypassed by vein grafts from the aorta.

SUMMARY

- Clogging of the arteries can in some cases be so severe that immediate measures to unclog them are necessary.
- One measure is surgery with plaque removal under direct vision (endarterectomy)—this is usually used for the carotid arteries.
- Other measures include squashing plaques with an inflated balloon (angioplasty) followed by insertion of a wire basket (stenting). Angioplasty and stenting are commonly used in the coronary arteries.
- Drugs can be used to unclog the arteries but may take several months to be effective; surgery and mechanical devices are used for urgent treatment when there are symptoms and a significant risk of heart attack or stroke.
- Other drugs (clot-busters) can be injected to dissolve thrombi at the site of a ruptured plaque. These have been successful in the early stages of heart attack but immediate angioplasty and stenting is generally preferable if the facilities are available.

Part VI

Targeted Groups

Some groups in the community have special
needs and need to be treated somewhat
differently—children, the elderly and pregnant
women are obvious examples.

34
Unclogging Women's Arteries

Some women tend to be a bit too complacent about their cardiovascular health as there is a popular belief that heart attack and stroke are predominantly diseases of men. Women perceive themselves to be more or less exempt.

This 'gender gap' in both popular belief as well as medical treatment is partly true because clogging of the arteries is certainly less common in women than men. But this applies only to premenopausal women. In fact, clogging of the arteries in women is a very important issue.

Once women reach menopause, they too are at cardio risk. An easy way to think of this is to remember that symptoms of clogging of the arteries occur about ten years later in women than men. Eventually, however, women do catch up—but not until the eighties. And since we are an ageing population, and many women will live well into their eighties, this is a serious health issue.

Some years ago I gave a presentation to an international women's medical conference on the topic of the 'gender gap' and its effect in getting women admitted into coronary care. My researches suggested that men were more likely than women to get into CCU (for intensive monitoring and treatment) even though both were eventually found to have suffered from heart attack. My presentation was one of the world's first in the area, and has been confirmed by later studies.

Lots of early research on clogging of the arteries looked only at men, because it was more difficult to get enough women to meet the statistical needs of the studies. Recently, however, women have been included in sufficient numbers to get a very good scientific basis for recommending treatment on the basis of evidence-based medicine. We'll learn more about these studies in this chapter.

Heart attacks in women

For many years, it has been recognised that heart attack rates in premenopausal women are significantly lower than in men of the same age. This difference becomes less after the menopause (age 50–55 years) until eventually heart attack rates become similar in elderly men and women over the age of 75 years.

Clogging of the arteries is less severe in younger women than men

I was once involved in a study of 50 men and 50 women, aged 50–55, who needed coronary angiography to see if clogging of the coronary arteries was responsible for their chest pain.

We saw that clogging of the arteries was more extensive in men than in women, affected more arterial segments, and was more severe. The average coronary score (which measured severity) was 14 in men and 9 in women. A completely blocked artery scored 4 points, 75–99 per cent narrowing scored 3 points, 50–74 per cent narrowing scored 2 points, and less than 50 per cent narrowing scored 1 point.

The protective effects of female hormones

The protection of younger women from heart attack has been attributed to hormonal differences between men and women, as well

as lifestyle factors. The hormone profile of women shows:
- Very low levels of the male hormone testosterone.
- High levels of the female hormones (oestrogens and progesterones).

These hormone differences can partly explain why men have lower HDL levels than women. Testosterone lowers HDL levels, and oestrogens raise them. Some progesterones raise HDL, while others lower HDL.

The lack of oestrogens in postmenopausal women may lower HDL levels slightly, and can have other detrimental effects, including loss of the normal protection of endothelial cells and a reduced capacity of arteries to dilate. Both factors may increase the risk of heart attack and stroke.

Trials of cholesterol-lowering drugs in women

In premenopausal years, women are at considerably lower risk of cardiovascular disease than men of the same age. After the menopause, however, the rate of cardiovascular disease in women increases and becomes almost as high as men, especially in the 'old elderly' over age 80. Most of the available evidence in women, as in the elderly, has been derived therefore from subgroup analysis of trials, which for the most part comprised middle-aged men. This evidence suggests, nevertheless, that lowering cholesterol benefits both men and postmenopausal women equally.

The Heart Protection Study

The clearest evidence to date has come from the Heart Protection Study. This was designed to include a large number of women at relatively high risk of heart attack. Over 5000 women were eventually included, who had either diabetes, high blood pressure or previous cardiovascular disease (see Table 34.1).

Table 34.1. Results of the Heart Protection Study.

Gender	Number	CV events Statin (%)	CV events Placebo (%)	per cent difference	NNT*
Men	15454	21.6	27.6	21.8	17
Women	5082	14.4	17.7	18.7	30

* NNT refers to the number of men and women needed to treat to prevent one event over the duration of the study.

The rate of cardiovascular events was significantly higher in placebo-treated than simvastatin-treated groups for both men and women. Event rates were also higher in men for both treatment groups. To prevent one event, 17 men needed to be treated with simvastatin for five years, compared with 30 women. This trial showed that cholesterol control in women with statins is beneficial in lowering cardiovascular disease events, including heart attack, coronary bypass and angioplasty as well as stroke.

SUMMARY

- Premenopausal women have a lower rate of cardiovascular disease than men.
- After the menopause, women catch up with men when they reach their late seventies.
- Risk factors apply equally to women and men with the exception of diabetes, which is more dangerous in women than men.
- HRT is no longer used to prevent cardiovascular disease in women older than 60.
- Statins lower cardiovascular disease rates as effectively in women as in men.

35
Unclogging Children's Arteries

We worry about our children all the time. But very few parents ever think about heart disease or clogged arteries in relation to their children. As a rule, children with high cholesterol issues go largely unrecognised, unless they have blood tests as part of a family screening program. This usually happens when a close relative has been found to have high cholesterol and the doctor suggests it might be a good idea to look at the rest of the family in order to pick up any potential problems at the earliest possible stage.

Other than through family testing, high cholesterol is detected in children on the rare occasions when cholesterol is so high that it causes skin, eye or tendon deposits. These are noted by the parents or by the family doctor on a routine visit. High triglycerides are uncommon in children and usually show up after puberty.

Children with high cholesterol may need to be treated at an early stage in order to prevent serious problems, some of which can occur quite early in adulthood.

Two groups of children need treatment. The first has high LDL of *polygenic* origin that responds well to dietary change. Many genes in these children are responsible for their high LDL levels, rather like height and weight. High LDL levels (also like height and weight) are passed down from one generation to the next. High LDL of polygenic origin is not very severe, and cholesterol levels are usually less than 7.0.

The other group does not respond to dietary change and has high LDL of *monogenic* origin. This means a single abnormal gene is responsible. As we discussed in the chapter on genetic disorders, these children suffer from one of two conditions: familial hypercholesterolaemia (FH) or familial defective apoB (FDB). Cholesterol levels are often higher than 7.0.

Children with FH and FDB are usually started on a cholesterol-lowering diet after the age of two. Many studies have shown no effects of such a diet on growth, development, intelligence or any measured variable. The best approach is for the whole family to go on the same diet, so the child does not feel they are being treated differently.

Drugs to lower LDL in children with FH or FDB are usually started after the age of ten years, and then only in severe cases in whom there is a family history of very early cardiovascular disease, or LDL levels are particularly high (see Chapter 11 for more details). The child with the more common polygenic variety of elevated LDL does not usually require drugs to lower cholesterol.

In all children with high LDL, it is crucial to prevent cigarette smoking because the combination of smoking and high LDL causes greatly accelerated clogging of the arteries. In most children, attention to diet and exercise to help with weight control can also significantly improve cholesterol levels, as for adults.

SUMMARY

- Blood fats in children should be checked if there is a family history of early-onset heart attack or stroke, or if there is a near relative with high cholesterol or triglycerides.
- High cholesterol or triglycerides can be from genetic causes or from such factors as overweight, low thyroid activity, and other diseases (as in adults).
- Severely elevated LDL levels in children can be treated with diet from the age of two years, and drugs as well as diet from the age of ten years.
- Children with high LDL levels must avoid cigarette smoking.
- Attention to diet and weight control can significantly improve cholesterol levels in many children (as in adults).
- Drugs are reserved for children with very high LDL and/or very early family history of cardiovascular disease.
- Statin treatment of children with genetic high LDL has been shown to prevent thickening of the carotid arteries over a 24-month period. Better results are obtained with earlier treatment, suggesting that children with this type of high LDL should be treated from the age of 10 years onwards.
- Children with genetic high LDL can be routinely diagnosed at the time of immunisation, when a blood test can also be taken. Since children have frequent visits to the doctor for immunisations, there is ample opportunity to perform screening tests for genetic high cholesterol. If a child is found to have high LDL, it is a simple matter to also measure LDL levels in both parents.

36
Unclogging Arteries in the Elderly

Perceptions of age and ageing have changed radically in the past couple of generations. Today youth is anywhere from 15 to 50, and then we have 'middle' age for the rest of our lives—or at least for as long as we possibly can manage to get away with it!

I look back on my grandparents, in their old-fashioned, shapeless clothing, their short grey hair, rimless spectacles, their too-white false teeth and unfit bodies, and they seem to me now (and looked to me then), about 100 years old. They were, however, probably in their early fifties.

People seemed to age faster in those days. Youth only lasted until marriage, middle age finished at 40 and old age set in at 50—at the latest!

Today the baby-boomers have changed all that. They want to look, feel, dress, act and live the way they did in their late thirties, even when they are in their sixties. To do so successfully, of course, they need to have fit bodies, both internally and externally. Many take this seriously. You only have to go out for a walk in the morning to see all the 'middle'-aged power walkers, in their trendy sports clothing.

Sometimes it's hard to tell the difference between a 45-year-old and a 65-year-old. But this is a relatively new phenomenon. A doctor has to be careful when predicting the age of a new patient—it is no longer easy to tell at a quick glance!

But whether we dye our hair, go to the gym, jog, walk daily, practise yoga, visit the plastic surgeon or buy our clothing in youth-wear shops, we do age internally. One of my professors used to say to us: 'We don't just get grey hair on our heads.' The implication, of course, was that our organs and our arteries age, even if we manage to disguise or stave off the external signs of ageing.

Who are the 'elderly'?

In the past, the definition of 'elderly' applied to people over the age of 65 years. Many research studies of cardiovascular disease didn't include people in this age group because there was some concern about the reliability of illness statistics (for example, old people often have several diseases which may contribute to a particular episode or hospital admission).

There was also considerable doubt about the benefits of lowering cholesterol in the elderly. This resulted from studies showing a weaker relationship between cholesterol and heart attack in the elderly compared with younger ages. In fact, these results may have been misinterpreted for complicated statistical reasons. The present approach is to consider cholesterol equally important as a risk factor with advancing age.

The definition of the elderly has now changed as a result of increasing ageing of the population ('grey power' and 'granny power' are realities that politicians and economists now take seriously). An increasing number of people are fit and active over the age of 80. There is a common and incorrect belief, for example, that most people of this age are in nursing homes. Quite the opposite is true. Most of the 'very old' are active, largely self-supporting, and living independently.

Attitudes to ageing are also changing. Fewer people are willing to accept the inevitability of growing old as a passive process over which we have no control. Like other, younger, age groups, the elderly are more interested in prolonging their health and taking more responsibility for it than ever before.

We now have a lot of information about the health benefits of lowering cholesterol (as well as blood pressure) in the elderly.

Cholesterol lowering with statins in the elderly

Previous results of cholesterol lowering in the elderly have been obtained from largely middle-aged populations that have included small numbers of subjects aged between 65 and 75 years. For example, a trial in the US with the drug lovastatin included 21 per cent aged over 65 (over 1330 elderly subjects), a trial in Scandinavia with simvastatin included 23 per cent (over 1000 subjects), a trial in the US with pravastatin included 31 per cent (over 1200), and a study in Australia and New Zealand with pravastatin included 31 per cent (over 3500).

These statin trials showed that the benefits from lowering rates of heart attack and stroke were similar in elderly and younger subjects.

The Heart Protection Study

The results of earlier statin trials were encouraging enough for the investigators of the recent Heart Protection Study (HPS) to include a large number of elderly people in their study. The results were conclusive. Cholesterol lowering with simvastatin resulted in significantly fewer heart attacks, deaths, bypass operations and strokes compared with a placebo-treated group. The results are shown in Table 36.1.

Table 36.1. Results of the Heart Protection Study.

Age	Number	per cent events* simvastatin	per cent events placebo	per cent placebo
< 65	9839	16.9	22.1	23.5
65-69	4891	20.9	27.2	23.2
70+	5086	23.6	28.7	17.8

* Events included heart attacks, strokes and revascularisation procedures (coronary bypass operations and balloon angioplasties)

The PROSPER Study

Another clinical trial of a statin to lower cholesterol in the elderly was the Prospective Study of Pravastatin in the Elderly at Risk (PROSPER) trial. This included 2804 men and 3000 women aged 70 to 82 years with a history of, or risk factors for, heart attack and stroke. They were treated for three years with either pravastatin (40 mg daily) or placebo. There were significant benefits of pravastatin treatment for a variety of cardiovascular diseases:

- Heart attacks: 19 per cent reduction
- Transient ischaemic attacks: 25 per cent reduction
- Heart attack and stroke: 15 per cent reduction

There were some unexpected results of the PROSPER trial, including no improvement in stroke rates nor intellectual functioning. (Some previous studies had suggested improvement in intellectual functioning with statin treatment in the elderly.) A small, non–significant increase in new cancers occurred in the pravastatin group (8.5 per cent versus 6.8 per cent in the placebo group); both rates were lower than predicted, however. All other statin trials have shown no effect on cancer rates.

Current recommendations

In the US, current recommendations are for cholesterol control in the elderly to be no different from younger people, although such factors as general health and functional ability should be taken into account when using drug treatment to lower cholesterol in older patients.

When an elderly person is found to have a high blood cholesterol level, it is very important to exclude other diseases which may have caused these high levels. Low thyroid activity is particularly important, because it is more common in the elderly and replacement of thyroid hormones is likely to cure the underlying disease as well as the high cholesterol.

SUMMARY

- The elderly are at high risk of heart attack and stroke.
- Lowering cholesterol with statins in the elderly can lower rates of death, heart attack and stroke, and can result in similar benefits to younger people.
- Age is no bar to treatment of high blood cholesterol.

37

Unclogging the Arteries after Heart Attack or Surgery

We've talked a lot about medications and the chemical warfare of cholesterol and triglyceride control in Part IV. But there is another very active front.

These days, there are some very successful and well-tolerated surgical procedures that restore blood supply to areas affected by clogging of the arteries, and which are performed often.

Surgeons are coming up with new techniques all the time, and refining existing techniques so that they are less invasive and take less toll on the patient, who in some cases can even go home the same day or the next.

The surgical teams are highly experienced and work together like one precise and modern machine. It is a privilege to be in the operating theatre to watch such procedures.

These 'surgical solutions' include coronary bypass operations, as well as bypass operations involving the carotid arteries and arteries to the legs and abdomen. Coronary angioplasty and stenting are performed more frequently than coronary bypass, and advances in technology have allowed cardiologists to stent more difficult lesions and multiple rather than single vessels.

Therefore, more and more people need cholesterol and triglyceride control following these revascularisation procedures. Once they have had the procedure, it is more critical than ever for them to have optimal control of *all* blood fats.

Survival after heart attack

Of 100 people suffering from a heart attack, about 30 die before reaching hospital. Most of these deaths occur within one hour of the first symptoms of chest pain or feeling unwell, and are usually caused by acute electrical instability of the heart, resulting in a very rapid heartbeat of about 300 per minute (the average heart rate at rest is 70–80 beats per minute). This rapid heartbeat (ventricular fibrillation) cannot sustain the blood flow to the body and is lethal within a few minutes. Underlying the sudden electrical instability is occlusion to coronary blood supply due to a ruptured atherosclerotic plaque (see Chapter 5).

The two-thirds of people surviving the first hour after onset of symptoms usually get to hospital, of whom 10–15 die during their hospital stay. Of those who make it out of hospital, a further 5–10 die in the first year, usually within the first two months after discharge. About 60 per cent of these early deaths after a heart attack occur suddenly.

The annual death rate after the first year is about 2–4 per cent but depends on age, other risk factors (such as smoking), the size of the initial heart attack, the site and severity of underlying coronary artery disease, and whether the patient is taking drugs such as aspirin, beta-blockers and statins. Long-term survival is higher in younger people, in whom the average five-year death rate is about 10 per cent below age 64 and about 45 per cent aged over 75.

People with small heart attacks, in which a small amount of heart muscle dies as a result of lack of blood supply, have a much better survival rate than those in whom large amounts of heart muscle die. The reason for this difference is probably related to the heart muscle's function as a pump. Damage to the heart muscle reduces its capacity to act as a pump, and heart failure may occur as a complication. Another reason why large heart attacks are more lethal is because they are associated with a higher rate of ventricular fibrillation, which is lethal unless resuscitation equipment is available.

What determines survival?

Having survived a heart attack, the major factor that determines long-term survival is the size of the heart attack. People with small heart attacks have up to five times better survival rates after five years than those with large heart attacks.

Another important factor is cigarette smoking. People who give up cigarettes have about half the heart attack rate of those who continue to smoke after a heart attack. The effectiveness of stopping smoking is even greater than that of drugs commonly used to improve survival. Drugs that increase survival include:

- Beta-blockers (which reduce the response of the heart to adrenaline).
- Angiotensin converting enzyme inhibitors or ACE inhibitors (which lower blood pressure and prevent dilatation of the heart).
- Aspirin (an anti-thrombotic drug that reduces platelet activity and 'thins the blood').
- Statins (which lower cholesterol; see Chapter 29).

Each of these drugs improves five-year survival by 20–30 per cent after heart attack. When added together, one can expect a reduction in heart attack rates by up to 80 per cent.

Several studies have shown that the risk of a second heart attack is greater in men with high cholesterol and LDL levels compared with men with low cholesterol and LDL levels. Other risk factors also affect survival rates. Those 10 per cent at lowest risk have more than a 90 per cent chance of survival after one year, have suffered very small heart attacks, are not smoking, have the lowest cholesterol, LDL and triglyceride levels, and have relatively normal electrocardiograms.

Following a heart attack, it is important that patients have their blood levels of cholesterol, HDL, LDL and triglycerides routinely measured. Those below the age of 60 may have a genetic form of high cholesterol. If LDL and/or triglyceride levels are high, or HDL levels are low, their children and close relatives should also have their levels measured. In this way, doctors can detect inherited disorders of cholesterol at a relatively early age, allowing them to measure other coronary risk factors and treat them at a time when control is most likely to halt or reduce the progression of clogging of the arteries.

People who've had coronary angioplasty, coronary stenting or coronary bypass surgery represent special groups who would also benefit from cholesterol and triglyceride control.

Many of these people have not suffered from a heart attack but rather from the earlier symptoms of coronary heart disease: angina.

Recent studies of bypassed coronary arteries and of the veins used for bypassing the coronary arteries have shown that clogging of the arteries in those that have been bypassed may rapidly worsen, and that clogging of the arteries may also affect the veins themselves. Clogging of the arteries in those used for bypass is usually much less severe, and the long-term results for arterial grafts are much better than vein grafts.

It is now apparent that long-term survival after this operation depends on the degree of clogging of the arteries of both the vein grafts and the coronary arteries. Between five and ten years after the operation, vein graft clogging of the arteries is a major cause for the development of symptoms requiring a second operation.

As would be expected from the way in which clogging of the arteries develops in arteries, clogging of the arteries in grafted veins is also related to blood cholesterol levels. Vein graft blockages occur earlier and more frequently in people with high cholesterol levels, as well as those with high triglyceride levels.

Studies of repeat coronary angiograms after bypass surgery have related the rate of narrowing of vein grafts to blood cholesterol and triglyceride levels. Average cholesterol and triglyceride levels have been higher in patients whose vein grafts showed progression after surgery than those with no progression.

In one study, people after coronary bypass surgery were randomised to treatment to achieve two levels of treatment with the statin, lovastatin. 'Aggressive' treatment lowered LDL levels to an average of 2.4, and was associated with less clogging of the arteries than 'moderate' treatment to achieve an average LDL level of 3.5.

SUMMARY

- Control of LDL and triglyceride levels is an important part of the routine management of patients after balloon angioplasty, stenting and coronary bypass surgery. This will reduce the rate of re-blocking after angioplasty, as well as clogging of vein grafts and arteries. It will also improve survival and delay the requirement, if any, for a second procedure.
- Current recommendations are to achieve the following levels:
  - Triglycerides less than 1.5
  - LDL less than 2.0
  - HDL more than 1.0
- Statin treatment is most frequently used to achieve these levels.

Part VII

Low-Chol Cuisine

By Marina Hamilton-Craig

The one thing I had not been groomed for
in childhood was to become the wife of a
cardiologist! My cooking methods and styles
have changed radically to incorporate
our low-cholesterol lifestyle.
Here are some of our favourite recipes.

Changing old habits

From the very beginning of my life with Ian, my Austro-Hungarian cooking methods needed to be totally revised and my cooking style radically changed. Out had to go the high-fat, high-cholesterol ingredients and in had to come a whole new attitude to food shopping, cooking, preparation and presentation.

My favourite handwritten recipes, passed down through several generations of my family, were precious to me and I did not want to completely pack them away, so I had to revise and rethink some of these family favourites to come up with food that was low-fat, low-chol, but high in flavour and presentation.

This was quite a challenge but eventually after numerous disasters I managed to evolve a new repertoire of truly healthy, usually interesting and sometimes gourmet dishes.

The most important thing I learnt was not to compromise on quality. This is vital.

If you can't use cream or butter or cheeses or pastry or other fats and hidden sugars such as in brandy or rum to mask or boost the flavour of a dish, you cannot use poor quality meat, fish, vegetables or fruit. You absolutely have to use the freshest and the best, because without all those disguising ingredients you will be very conscious of the basic flavours.

The best cuts are, of course, the most expensive cuts, so I learnt to cook like an Italian housewife—little amounts and fine slices of fish or meat, of the very best quality, backed up with the freshest vegetables, cooked lightly to be slightly *al dente*, as they were not going to be covered with a thick layer of buttery sauce.

I learnt to use tiny new potatoes instead of large, floury ones, so there was no need for salt, pepper, butter and sour cream with chives to disguise the slightly musty flavour of the vegetable. Instead you could actually taste the potato, enhanced with perhaps just a sprinkling of fresh chives or parsley. (If you love the creamy texture of sour cream, try low-fat yoghurt instead.) I made friends with spices. Not the sorts you get in jars or packages, but the sort you grind yourself, and which fill your kitchen with their delicious, tantalising aromas.

I grew familiar with the fish markets and the stall-keepers and learnt how to scale, fillet and slice fish. The stall-keepers showed me how to recognise the freshest fish (clear eyes) and how to settle for nothing less.

Finally, I began to recognise the true sophistication of simplicity, and that *haute cuisine* in this era is about fresh, top quality food which tastes of itself.

This is not the *cucina povera* of minimal amounts of fruit and vegetables and the worst cuts of grisly meat, covered with thick, heavy pastry, served with dumplings or boosted with mashes and sauces to make them go further and to disguise their lack of freshness or their intrinsic toughness. You know the sort of dishes I mean—things like toad-in-hole, or apple dumplings or bread-and-butter pudding, which are all just ways of stretching the rations and filling hungry tummies for minimal cost.

This was the cuisine of cold countries in the times before air-conditioning and electric/gas heating. It was of the era when food needed to fuel you on the two-mile walk to work in the drizzling rain. It was the cuisine of the farmer's wife who had to feed many on few rations. It is not the food we need today.

Today we live in a society where fresh food is plentiful and still relatively inexpensive, where we drive to work, sit at desks, and have heated homes. We can afford to eat well if we shop selectively and go to farmers' markets to get fresh food at low prices. Also, if you buy good quality there is little waste and you use all you pay for—no bones and fat to cut off and discard. I have learnt to make the most of it all.

So I threw out my old ideas of apple pies, which were all pastry with a few slivers of apple in the centre, drowned in sugar and packed in huge amounts of fat-filled white flour pastry. Instead I learnt to make pastry-free pies with layers of baked apple sprinkled with fresh ginger and crushed cinnamon stick and sweetened—not always necessary—with a light sprinkling of dried currants and baked until just golden brown.

Instead of cream I found I could serve them with low-fat ricotta, whipped up with skimmed milk and dusted with a fine coating of nutmeg.

Added benefits were we slept better because our stomachs were not overfilled before bedtime, and so we felt like going for a walk after dinner with the dog. We were not as sleepy as we had been, as our bodies were not overloaded with those heavy, difficult-to-digest meals that make you lie in bed feeling like a beached whale. We actually felt better. I lost weight without even trying and our low-chol cuisine became an established part of our lives.

Other than fresh herbs, which I like to grow myself, my other new best friends in the kitchen have become dry red and white wine. While the high sugar brandy-cream sauces of my past were shelved forever, red and white dry wines began to appear regularly not only on the table but in the actual food.

Ours has become a Mediterranean diet.

A rich vegetable soup for example, not unlike a minestrone, is a favourite first course, served with crusty bread and a touch of olive oil, followed by a grilled or baked fish, meat or chicken dish, served with a green salad or one single green vegetable such as beans, snowpeas or broccoli, and finally finished with a large bowl of seasonal fresh fruit. I love in-season fruit which tastes of the season—crisp autumn apples, summer peaches, winter mandarins.

A fruit platter is a veritable feast, and one that lends itself to endless combinations.

Breakfast

I once read a book which said one should breakfast like a king, lunch like a prince and dine at night like a pauper. There is no doubt this is a good way to eat, as you have your energy when you need it most.

It is hard to put into practice when you are living a busy life. We tend to do this more on weekends—a big breakfast, a late lunch and a light dinner. Certainly I always sleep well when we eat like this.

Otherwise we tend to have a solid breakfast, a light lunch and when possible an early but substantial dinner.

Porridge

Ian is a great a believer in oats—perhaps because of his Scottish background. Oats, in particular oat bran, have a cholesterol-lowering effect although you have to eat a huge amount of oats to make a difference, but there is still no doubt that the oat is a wonder food, good for digestion, good for body-building and can keep you going for a long and busy day. Don't just put milk on it, be creative with flavour-enhacing fruit and nuts.

1 cup of oats
2 cups of water
Skimmed milk
Apple, grated
Dried fruit (apricots, prunes, apples, peaches)
chopped nuts
Banana or strawberries, sliced
Low-fat yoghurt
Cinnamon

Combine the oats and water. Use a deep bowl if microwaving, or place in small saucepan on stove top. You can vary the ratio to suit yourself. More water makes a creamier porridge. I use boiling water to hurry the process along, but if you have time cold water is slower and the result is better! Cook in microwave on about 50 per cent heat for 3–4 minutes, or heat in saucepan until it thickens.

While cooking add grated apple, or dried fruits.

When oats have thickened, you can create your own bowl. Serve with skimmed milk (or not), sliced fresh fruit such as banana or strawberry, and chopped nuts. Top with a dash of yoghurt and/or sprinkled cinnamon.

Homemade toasted muesli

Because we live in a warm climate we have homemade muesli for breakfast for about nine months of the year and porridge for three. Make up a big batch which can last for two to three weeks. Quantities vary according to your own taste.

Oats (plain or toasted)
Sugar-free processed bran
Oat bran
Wholewheat breakfast biscuit cereal
Dried fruit
Chopped nuts (almonds)
Seeds (pumpkin, sunflower)

If you prefer toasted muesli, toast the oats on a flat tray on a low temperature oven for approximately 20 minutes (stir them around half way through and don't forget them—they will burn). Toast chopped almonds in the same way. Add sugar-free processed bran, oat bran, crumbled wholewheat breakfast biscuit cereal, dried currants, dried apple and oven-roasted chopped almonds.

Serve with skimmed milk, plain homemade yoghurt (see below) and on weekends with tropical fruits such as kiwis, mangos, strawberries and pawpaw. On weekdays we just unzip a banana.

Use this muesli as a crumble for pudding or fruit salad with yoghurt.

Hot breakfasts

Baked beans on toast, sprinkled with fresh parsley
Canned corn, served with toast or made into an egg white omelet.
Grilled tomatoes on toast
Swiss mushrooms, oven-baked and served on wholemeal toast.

Eggs

Limiting your intake of egg yolks will decrease your fat and cholesterol consumption. I very occasionally make French toast using just egg white, but that is a Sunday or special occasion such as a birthday or Father's Day treat!

The other big family treat—and I always do this for Easter Sunday—is wholemeal pancakes made again using only egg whites—and served with real maple syrup, grilled banana, fresh blueberries and yoghurt. Bliss!

Yoghurt

I make my own yoghurt—the easy way—with a home yoghurt kit, where you just add water to the powder and leave overnight in a warm water bath. You can get fat-free powder. I have one jar in the fridge and one developing every second day. We go through a lot and this method is so quick and easy!

Of course buying yoghurt is easy, too. Get the best quality, with plenty of acidophilus, to keep your insides healthy.

Nibbles

Smoked salmon

Smoked salmon, on very thin brown bread with a scraping of horse-radish, and topped by paper-thin lemon slices. Hard to beat with a glass of dry white wine for a meal starter.

Olive oil and balsamic vinegar

Virgin olive oil, mixed with a bit of balsamic vinegar and used as a dip for crusty brown bread. Dead easy and rather smart!

Dukkah

I make my own dukkah, full of very acceptable low-chol goodies:

150g shelled and toasted hazelnuts
150g lightly toasted almonds (with skins)
50g toasted sesame seeds
50g toasted coriander seeds
50g cumin powder

Put all ingredients into a food processor and process until the consistency of rough sand. Do not over-process, otherwise the oils are released by the nuts and make the mixture 'wet'.

Serve in a dish and put out identical dishes of extra virgin olive oil and balsamic vinegar for people to dip into with crusty wholemeal bread. A great dinner starter and ideal for vegetarians.

Sprinkle dukkah on firm flesh fish before baking it to get a nice, flavoursome crust. You can also do this with baked chicken pieces, making a sort of Middle Eastern chicken Maryland!

Tuna pate

The very word pate makes cholesterol experts shudder, but here is one which is totally OK:

1 can tuna in spring water, drained
1 tablespoon fat-free mayonnaise
rind of half a lemon
juice of half a lemon
dash of chilli sauce (optional)

Throw all the ingredients into the food processor and blend until you get a smooth paste (or pate). Serve with fresh wholemeal toast or pieces of crudites such as carrot and zucchini rounds, and sprinkle with dill. You can add dill to the pate for extra flavour.

You can reserve the tuna juice and sprinkle in a packet of gelatine (about a dessert spoon) and then blend with the tuna mixture and allow to set and turn out for a pate you can slice with a knife. When I am doing a dinner party I sometimes made individual moulds, but it is easier to serve individual dishes, such as those tiny Asian cups used for green teas.

If I am really going all out, I made a sauce of two tablespoons of fat-free mayonnaise mixed with about a centimetre of wasabi sauce from a tube. This not only makes a pretty pale green colour but is a great topping for the tuna pate.

Yes, you can use pink salmon instead if you like.

'Pastry' cases

Pastry is a no-no on the low-chol scene, but I make nice little 'pastry' cases out of day-old sliced bread, cut into squares and flattened into muffin tin holes, and baked to just golden in a medium oven.

These cases are great for various fillings. My favourites include:

Slices of fresh raw tuna topped with the wasabi mayonnaise above
Tuna pate with lemon slices
Pink beef topped with French mustard
Pink lamb topped with mint jelly

Hungarian paprika spread

This is a dish of my youth, with the cream and butter left out. It's an ideal dip, and also great served with triangles of toast as a starter.

1 cup low-fat cottage cheese
1 tablespoon sweet paprika (less if you prefer) but it must
be fresh and orange in colour
1 teaspoon French mustard
1 tablespoon chopped chives (optional)
2 tablespoons low-fat yoghurt

Chuck it all in the blender or food processor and mix. Some people add caraway seeds, but I don't like them.

You can make it a bit 'hotter' by adding a tiny bit of cayenne pepper if you like. I also like this on top of baked potatoes.

Vegetable Dishes

Vegetables don't have cholesterol, so are a great way to keep your food intake healthy. Here are a few of my tried-and-true favourites. You can vary most of them to broaden your repertoire.

Butternut pumpkin shell

1 medium-sized butternut pumpkin
1 tablespoon onion flakes, browned in Teflon pan
1 cup steamed brown rice
2 tablespoons chopped fresh sage or basil
Cayenne pepper to taste
Chopped parsley

Cut the pumpkin through the middle lengthwise and clean out the central hole. Stuff with mixtures of rice, sage and onion, moistened with a dash of vegetable stock or water, just enough to make it slightly sticky. Loosely cover with foil and bake in low oven until pumpkin is cooked—soft through when tested with a sharp knife or skewer. (If you are in a hurry you can 'prep' the pumpkin without the filling by cooking in microwave at 50 per cent heat for four minutes.)

Serve on a bed of steamed baby spinach leaves and sprinkled with chopped parsley.

A nice sauce for this is bottled tomato and basil pasta sauce, served warm in a jug. Too easy!

Greek stuffed tomatoes

This is a simplified version of a classic recipe and makes a great lunch dish served with lightly steamed greens such as baby spinach or with a mixed green salad. You really need to make this in summer when big, red tomatoes are in season—pale tomatoes just don't have enough flavour.

Four slices of fresh, thinly sliced wholemeal bread
4 large ripe cooking tomatoes
1 onion or a tablespoon of dried onion flakes
2 teaspoons chopped fresh thyme (or 1 teaspoon dried thyme)
2 cups cooked brown rice
Olive oil

Take four ramekins or small ovenproof soufflé dishes, about the size of a large teacup. Cut the bread into rounds, using the dish as a cutter. Remove the top quarter of the tomato and place in the oven-proof dish (use top of the tomato in the salad if you like). Scoop out the centre of the tomato and mix the tomato pulp with the chopped onion, rice and herbs and fill the tomato cases. Bake lightly covered in slow to moderate oven for 20 minutes or until tomato is cooked but not mushy. Then place a bread round, brushed lightly with olive oil, over each tomato, and continue to bake until bread is toasted to a nice, golden brown.

This makes a great main dish or vegetable to go with meat or fish, as well as a nice little entrée or luncheon dish. A sprig of fresh thyme on top is the gourmet touch.

You can also use a small eggplant or aubergine instead of tomato. You may need to cook it a little longer.

Or replace the tomato with a small golden nugget pumpkin—scoop out and discard the seeds and use 2 cups of rice, spiced with a touch of nutmeg. Replace the top or 'hat' of the pumpkin and bake. This might take a bit longer, perhaps 30 minutes. Test with a skewer after about 25 minutes.

Stuffed capsicums

This is a classic Hungarian dish known as stuffed paprika or stuffed capsicum, adapted to Ian's eating rules.

2 large red and 2 green capsicums
500g lean topside mince
1 cup of cold cooked brown rice
½ cup chopped onion
2 cans peeled tomatoes
Handful chopped parsley

Cut capsicums in half and remove pith and seeds, creating empty cups. Mix meat, cooked rice, parsley, chopped onions and season with a touch of black pepper (personally I prefer not to use pepper, but you may like a touch).

Make meat mixture into large balls and press into capsicum caps. Stand cups in baking dish, and pour over tomato sauce made by blending peeled tomatoes until smooth (or you can use a bottle of tomato-and-basil *sugo* or even a can of condensed tomato soup, if you are in a hurry).

Make sure you have enough liquid to reach almost to the top of the cups. Cover and bake slowly for about an hour, or until capsicum is soft but still holding its shape. Serve with rice, pasta or steamed potato, or just with a green salad.

The flavour from the two colours of capsicum seeps into the sauce, making it into a unique Hungarian dish. If you like you can sprinkle paprika powder and parsley on your accompanying potato/rice/pasta for an authentic touch. This dish can be made the day before and gently heated, but it takes a while for the heat to get through to the centre of the meatball, so give it plenty of time. I like it best fresh, of course.

Stuffed mushrooms

Use the same ingredients as for Stuffed capsicums, but use very large Swiss brown mushrooms, adding chopped mushroom stems into the filling mixture. Bake for a shorter time, perhaps 20 to 30 minutes, depending on the size of the mushroom. I sometimes use a can or two of undiluted, low-salt mushroom soup instead of the tomato for this dish, which gives it quite a rich, creamy taste.

Not-nasty vegetable pasties

Place a shop-bought pasty on a piece of paper and just see the fat seeping out. Not a good look! You can make your own fat-free vegetable pasty with just as much flavour. You can vary the amounts below to suit your taste.

Three sheets of filo pastry, each brushed with beaten egg white
Cubed potato, carrot, parsnip, pumpkin
Chopped cabbage
Onion
Homemade tomato sauce

Steam the vegetables until just done. Steam chopped cabbage and lightly fried onion. Add black pepper to taste. Lay two sheets of pastry on top of each other. Cut into two triangles. Spoon filling on to each triangle and cover with remaining triangle. Fold edges over, bake on baking paper until pastry is golden brown. Serve with homemade tomato sauce.

Soups

Soups are a tasty way to start a meal, make a filling snack and a great lunch with crusty wholemeal bread. Here are a few of my favourite family soups. The quantities can vary according to taste. They work for two people or you can make a whole cauldron for a party.

Roast pumpkin and pea soup

Quarter of a pumpkin
1 large cooked potato, cubed
Low-salt vegetable cube
Handful of tiny frozen peas
Dollop of low-fat yoghurt
Fresh herbs to serve
Brown sugar (optional)

Use the best quality, bright orange pumpkin. Cut into pieces and microwave, until just barely tender. Cut off the skin (this is much easier to do than when it is raw). Pop into a hot oven on baking paper and bake until just starting to brown at the edges. In the meantime, microwave about half as much potato as the pumpkin you used.

Chuck the baked pumpkin and the potato into a blender, a little at a time and blend with one low-salt vegetable cube. Return to a saucepan and add boiling water a little at a time until you have the consistency you want. Add frozen peas a minute before serving so they just barely cook. Serve with a dollop of low-fat yoghurt and a sprinkling of any green fresh herb you like (basil, coriander, parsley, etc). I sometimes add a teaspoon of brown sugar, which brings out the pumpkin flavour.

Cauliflower bisque

Half a cauliflower
One large peeled potato cubed
1 cup low fat milk
Nutmeg to taste
2 cups real vegetable stock

Cut up cauliflower, leaving some of the light green tender leaves. Cook cauliflower and potato cubes in stock until just barely done. Puree in food processor and add milk to taste—usually you won't need a whole cup as this soup is best fairly thick. Add a dash of white pepper and served dusted with nutmeg.

Potato and corn chowder

2 cups cubed peeled potato
Dash of white pepper
1 cup corn kernels, cooked
1 cup skim milk

Simmer potato in a minimum of water until soft. Blend in food processor with a dash of white pepper and milk and add the cooked corn at the very last minute so it breaks up but does not puree. Serve this nice and thick. I sometimes reserve a bit of corn to use as a garnish on top.

Fish chowder

Follow the Potato and corn chowder recipe on the previous page and at the last minute add some fresh boneless white fish and let it cook for a few minutes, then break it up with a fork and blend it into the soup. For a party use a few prawns to add a touch of class! A half a cup or so of frozen peas adds colour and texture to this soup. In an emergency you can use tinned fish for this recipe but it is not quite as nice—a bit too fishy.

Carrot coriander soup

6 large peeled carrots diced
1 medium potato peeled and chopped
2 cups real vegetable stock
1 large onion peeled and chopped
Roasted coriander seedings, to garnish

Cook carrots, onion and cubed potato in the stock till soft. Puree in blender and season with white pepper. Add carefully washed chopped coriander at last moment and sprinkle with roasted coriander seeds for texture.

Everyone loves this soup. A variation is to use julienned orange zest instead of coriander. Blanch the skin of one orange, julienne the zest and add to soup at last minute. Decorate with a thin orange slice.

Parsnip and pear soup

As above but use parsnips instead of carrots and sliced fresh pear instead of coriander. I microwave the sliced pear for about 30 seconds.

Cheat minestrone

This is an absolute cheat recipe, but very handy to have in the pantry.

1 large packet real beef stock
1 packet low-salt French onion soup mix
1 tin three or four bean salad mix
1 tin peas and carrots
1 tin corn kernels
1 tin whole potatoes
1 packet 2-minute chicken noodles

Heat the stock with French onion soup mix; chuck in the carefully rinsed beans, peas and carrots. Add corn, juice and all. Slice the potato into cubes. Heat through. Add the noodles from the 2-minute noodle soup, without the flavouring, but crush to make noodles small. Heat through for 2 minutes and serve with hot crusty bread. This is so fast; you need to have the bread in the oven before you begin the soup! A sprinkling of Italian herb mix gives an authentic touch.

You can get away with all tins if you must, but if you have time, microwave your own potato and carrots to add, as it does taste more homemade.

Yes, a small sprinkling of Parmesan cheese is allowed, even by Ian—but only a bit!

Curried vegetable soup

1 packet of raw soup vegetables
2 cups real vegetable stock
1 dessert spoon of your favourite curry paste
3cm fresh ginger, grated
sprinkle of dessicated coconut

Peel and chop the vegies to all about the same size. Cook vegies in the stock and the fresh ginger, adding the curry paste about halfway through the cooking (at about 10 minutes). Sprinkle with a dusting of coconut before serving with freshly microwaved pappadams (much better than cooking them in oil) and a bowl of fresh natural low-fat yoghurt, sprinkled with chopped mint or dried mint from a jar as a last resort. You can add a couple of bits of hot chilli if you like your curries hot.

Main Courses

Steak

We like to have red meat occasionally but we tend to have the leanest cuts. I use fillet of beef seared on the outside and pink in the middle, sliced finely while it is warm and fanned out on the plate—you use less steak and somehow it is more digestible as well as working out not so expensive per person.

With steak, my favourite sauce is a tablespoon of honey melted in a fry pan, and when bubbling topped with half a cup of Balsamic vinegar and cooked until it is reduced a bit and poured over the steak, resting on baby spinach leaves. A family favourite, and certainly smart enough for a dinner party.

Spicy crust lamb cutlets

1 tablespoon coriander seeds
1 tablespoon cumin powder
1 tablespoon toasted sesame seeds
1 tablespoon chopped mint
1 cup low-fat yoghurt
8 French trimmed lamb cutlets (no visible fat)

Combine two spices and sesame seeds and press onto meat to coat. Lay on baking paper and bake in medium oven until cooked but pink in middle. Mix yoghurt with mint to make sauce. Serve meat on bed of couscous, made with Middle Eastern spices and a tablespoon of dried currants, sweated baby spinach leaves and a tablespoon of yoghurt mint sauce per serve.

Turkey

One of the underused foods of our time is turkey. Our old friend the turkey tends to appear at Christmas and perhaps Easter, but the rest of the year it seems to be off the menu.

Turkey is relatively low in fat and cholesterol. I tend to use fine slices of turkey breast where traditional recipes use veal. *Natur* (natural) schnitzel is merely slices of veal, pan-fried. You can do this with turkey in a nonstick pan with a minimum of fat such as a film of olive oil: Slice your meat thinly, coat in flour and then spread with grainy mustard. Cook lightly on both sides and serve with a sauce using the scrapings of the pan, bubbled up with a glass of white wine, and then poured over the meat. Wonderful with boiled new potatoes and the classic cucumber salad (finely sliced cucumber in vinaigrette or in plain yoghurt, topped with sprinkling of paprika).

Roast turkey drumsticks

One drumstick is sometimes enough for two people. Bake on a sheet of non-stick baking paper, surrounded by vegies of your choice. Any left-over drumstick makes a great pate, blended up with a few spices and a dash of BBQ sauce.

Baked turkey breast

1kg turkey breast without skin
Wholemeal bread/sage and onion stuffing, moistened with water
and a touch of olive oil.

Make a pocket in the meat and stuff with mixture. Seal with metal skewer. Bake on baking paper for 1 hour, basting frequently. Basting juice: Lightly fry one chopped onion in a nonstick pan; add chopped sage, juice and grated rind of one orange and a teaspoon of honey. Serve with parsnips, carrots, and potatoes baked in a separate dish, and also occasionally basted with basting mixture. A green salad really finishes off this dish. I sometimes use rosemary instead of sage.

Fish

Fish is Ian's preferred protein, so we eat a lot of it.

Poached salmon with mustard dill sauce

4 salmon fillets

1 tablespoon olive oil

1½ cups low-fat milk

1 dessertspoon cornflour

Juice of one small lemon

2 teaspoons French mustard

Chopped dill to taste

Parsley

Barely sear fish on both sides in olive oil. Add hot milk and turn down heat. Season with freshly ground pepper. Simmer until fish is done. Move fish to warm platter and cover. Mix cornflour and lemon juice in small bowl, add poaching liquid to fill bowl, stir and then transfer contents back to pan. Stir gently till beginning to thicken, add mustard and chopped parsley and dill to taste. Serve fish with mustard dill sauce and boiled new potatoes and peas.

Dukkah-crumbed fish

Take any firm-flesh fish, such as blue-eye cod, Atlantic salmon, ocean trout or similar and cut into two-centimetre finger serves. Coat with dukkah (see Nibbles) and bake on baking paper for about 12–15 minutes until done. Serve with fresh lime and give each person two fingers of fish. Great served over couscous, which complements the Middle Eastern mood of this dish.

Wasabi salmon

One fillet or cutlet of salmon per person
½ cup light soy sauce
1 teaspoon wasabi paste
½ cup water
3cm peeled fresh ginger, julienne or one teaspoon crushed ginger
2 bok choy per person, lightly steamed
steamed rice

Mix soy, wasabi, water and ginger in bowl and set aside. Cook fish until done—but not overcooked—in non stick pan, just barely smeared with olive oil. When fish is done serve on lightly steamed bok choy and steamed rice and drizzle over with the warmed soy mixture. (I sometimes make double the sauce as it is very popular with the family.)

Thai fish balls

500g white fish (any you like, without bones)
2 teaspoon crushed ginger
1 teaspoon lemongrass chopped
2 kaffir lime leaves, finely sliced
light soy sauce
¼ teaspoon hot chilli (optional)
1 egg white

Mash fish in blender and add other ingredients to just blend through. Form into flat patties and either bake or cook in non-stick fry pan. Serve with fresh lime, coconut rice and Asian steamed greens.

Pasta

It has often been said that the Mediterranean diet is ideal for those conscious of heart-smart eating. Well, you can't do Med unless you do pasta, can you?

My favourite is *spirali*, as it seems to collect the sauce best on all those surfaces, but Ian likes *tagliatelle* and our son loves *farfel* and my mother, once she mastered classic spaghetti twirling with a fork and spoon, always asked for that, to show off her skills. She could eat a bowlful without spilling a drop of sauce or missing a single noodle!

There are as many sauces as there are types of pasta—more, in fact— but to my mind there is nothing as good with pasta as a simple tomato *sugo* or sauce.

The best taste is fresh, sun-ripened, just-picked tomatoes. You can make this yourself or cheat by buying the best quality tomato-and-basil sauce in a jar, and adding quartered cherry tomatoes to 'freshen' up the sauce. Cherry tomatoes have more flavour than most of their larger siblings and the flavour just bursts through the sauce. I always have basil growing, with one pot coming along, another ready to harvest and one just planted. Can't live without basil!

Otherwise I love *al dente* pasta with nothing but extra virgin olive oil, a grinding of fresh pepper and a tiny bit of garlic. So simple but so wonderful! The Italians add salt, but Ian doesn't and I don't miss it. I sometimes add a bit of chopped rosemary, which is just heaven, lightly braised in olive oil and then poured over freshly cooked pasta.

Salads

You can put anything into a salad … meat, nuts, greens of course, fruit and even bread. But the main thing to remember is that a salad should be fresh, have texture and leave you feeling as if you have eaten something light, so don't overdo the ingredients or the dressing.

I still think the best salad to go with a meal (as opposed to a salad which is a meal) is an all green salad, made up of a variety of lettuces, baby spinach, a touch of rocket, some slices of avocado and a nice oil/vinegar/seed mustard dressing.

But of course there are all kinds of fancy meal-in-a-bowl salads.

The greatest of these has got to be salade nicoise, the famous fisherman's salad of the south of France.

Salade Nicoise

Salad greens
Wedges of ripe red tomato
Chunks of tuna (canned in spring water)
Slices of steamed potato (optional)
Anchovies
Black olives

Line a salad bowl with greens; add tomato, tuna and potato if you are using it. Lay strips of anchovy over the top, and sprinkle with black olives. Drizzle with your best oil/vinegar dressing. Serve with chunks of crusty bread. Yes, the traditional dish does have hardboiled egg in wedges. I sometimes use egg white in slices but not the yolk, which is too high in cholesterol. No-one has ever said they miss it!

Tomato and basil panzenella

4 slices day-old bread per serve
1 large Spanish onion, finely sliced into rings, and soaked in fresh water for
half an hour
4 large tomatoes per serve
1 small bunch basil, chopped
½ cup extra virgin olive oil
¼ cup balsamic vinegar
Kalamata olives
4 teaspoons lemon juice

Place one slice of bread with crusts removed into each salad bowl. Top with rinsed onion rings. Add finely sliced tomatoes, each layer topped with torn basil. Mix lemon juice, olive oil and vinegar and pour over each serving. Add touch of freshly ground pepper. Cover each bowl and set aside until serving time. This is best made about four hours ahead. Serve at room temperature, not cold.

Rocket and pear salad

My favourite salad green is rocket, which has a great, almost radishy taste.

Rinse your rocket and place in a bowl. Add paper-thin slices of fresh, firm pear and cover with your favourite vinaigrette dressing. Yes, some people do add slivers of Parmesan cheese to this salad—I sprinkle a few walnuts or pecan nuts instead. I promise it is just as good. Actually, I think it's better.

Baby spinach with water chestnuts

1 cup baby spinach leaves
1 cup bok choy, carefully washed and finely sliced
½ cup sliced water chestnuts
Vinaigrette dressing

Mix the greens, top with chestnuts and serve with dressing.

Waldorf salad

2 chopped red apples
2 chopped green apples
½ cup walnuts or pecan nuts
Creamy dressing made with low-fat yoghurt/mustard/chopped mint and
tiniest touch of honey (optional)

Mix all ingredients and serve in lettuce cups.

Beetroot salad

We have all begun to think that beetroot comes out of tins. Try using fresh beetroot and taste the difference.

Steam raw beetroot until just tender. Remove outer skin and slice or wedge. I prefer wedges as it does not look like the tinned kind. While still warm, put into a bath of 1 cup water, ½ cup vinegar and a teaspoon of sugar. Leave overnight. Drain and serve. Great with fish.

Margo's new potato salad

Peel and steam new potatoes. While warm, put into vinegar bath as above. Cool and let the spuds absorb the flavour. Then discard bath when cool. Serve drained potatoes with a dressing of yoghurt, seed mustard and mint. You can use fat-free mayonnaise instead of yoghurt. I sometimes use half mayo and half yoghurt. Some people prefer parsley to mint. Lots of people add onion, but I think it spoils the clean taste.

Puddings and Desserts

There is no dessert as good as fresh seasonal fruit. In my family, dessert means fruit and pudding is the term used for anything from ice-cream to Christmas plum pud.

In the warmer season, we always have fresh fruit to end the meal in our house. Put the fruit bowl and a bowl of water on the table and perhaps a bowl of nuts and let everyone do the washing, peeling and cracking for themselves.

Baked apples

In winter I sometimes create hot winter puds, such as baked apples filled with a mix of dried fruits and nuts.

A nice 'pie' is just slices of apple, sprinkled with ginger and nutmeg or cinnamon and baked, as previously mentioned. You can do the same with pears.

Bananas

I like bananas baked in orange juice and then sprinkled with spices and a few raisins. It's a great way of using up old bananas. You can also freeze bananas, skin and all, and then peel and toss into the blender with a bit of low-fat cottage cheese for a lovely banana mousse or crème.

Another great ice-cream style pud is frozen banana beaten up with a bit of lime juice and served in long-stemmed glasses with fresh strawberries on top.

Rhubarb

Steam rhubarb with a stick of cinnamon and a teaspoon of honey and serve with yoghurt or make into a crumble by serving with a sprinkling of homemade muesli and putting under the griller for a few seconds.

Dried fruit compote

In winter, a popular compote is mixed dried fruit, soaked overnight in black tea and then served warm with yoghurt. Very Middle Eastern and quite gourmet!

Mousse

I do have a great mousse or semifreddo as a party pud:

1 carton low-fat ice-cream
Juice and grated rind of a large orange
1 tablespoon Grand Marnier liqueur
1 packet gelatin

Soften the ice-cream and mix in all the ingredients. Take a dessert spoon of gelatin and soften in half a cup of warm water. Add to ice-cream mix and turn into a metal or plastic bowl and freeze overnight. Serve by dipping bowl in hot water and turning pud out onto a plate. You can make this in individual glasses and make life easy for yourself. Top with fresh red berries. Very smart and relatively healthy for party fare.

Apple crumble

Heat canned unsweetened pie apples in the microwave, sprinkle with cinnamon and top with home-made muesli (see breakfast). Best crumble you ever had and both fat-free and low in time and labour! Of course you can peel, slice and cook your own apples if you have time. You can do this trick with tinned apricot pie filling, or fresh rhubarb, pears or even tinned pineapple, or indeed any other fruit you like.

Strudel

You can make your own strudels with filo pastry, brushed with beaten egg white, and filled with drained bottled cherries or tinned pie apples, mixed with a small handful of dried currants. Layer a row of fruit on the pastry and fold over the edges and tuck in the ends and then bake on my favourite kitchen tool (baking paper!) until pastry is just light brown. Allow to cool and cut on the paper and serve or it will almost certainly break. Low fat ice-cream is nice with barely warm strudel.

I find a lot of low fat products are very high in sugar, so look at the labels before buying!

Appendix

Unclogging the Arteries: Past, Present and Future

As trainee cardiologists, my colleagues and I were aware of the huge advances being made in medications and both invasive and non-invasive medical imaging, testing and diagnosis. Our training was quite difficult and challenging and we used to joke that after all that study and work, it was likely that we'd all be back in 20 years, retraining as geriatricians, because within our working lifetime the need for cardiologists would diminish dramatically.

Well, as far as I am aware, none of my former colleagues have had to undertake such retraining, but we certainly have seen enormous changes in cardiology care since we began to practise.

When I wrote my first book on cholesterol, I made some predictions for cholesterol control in the 21st century, thinking of the 2020s to 2030s. We are only a short way into the 21st century, and some of my earlier and more important predictions have already come true. The pace of scientific development has been much faster than I imagined, and is likely to be even faster in the future.

In this chapter I'd like to review the original predictions, and make new ones to look back on in another 15 years' time! Let's look at these original predictions and comments:

1. *'Smoking cigarettes has become socially unacceptable and smoking in public is prohibited. No tobacco advertising is allowed. The tobacco companies have diversified and invested most of their capital into the clothing industry and land-based fish farms. Death rates from lung cancer begin to fall for the first time.'*

Fifteen years later (now): Most of these predictions have been fulfilled. We see non-smoking areas offices, public places, restaurants. Smoking in Western countries is certainly on the decline, especially among the well-educated and higher income groups. Smoking in teenagers (especially girls) is still increasing in spite of advertising bans. Hollywood is no help with the popularity of retro-movies.

Fifteen years from now: Smoking rooms are passé at airports, hotels and other public places because these are designated to be smoke-free zones. We joke abut the days when there used to be 'smoking' and non-smoking' areas and seats in aircraft, which were one row apart so non-smokers could breathe in side-stream smoke through the whole flight.

2. *'Gero-boy' and 'Gero-girl' become top-selling magazines, as the proportion of the geriatric population over 70 increases to more than 30 per cent. Retirement villages abound in all suburbs and in most large country towns. Many have their own private tennis courts, swimming pool, indoor gymnasium, jogging track and nine-hole golf courses. Gero-power is pervading society. Surrogate grannies and grandpas mind small children while their parents go to work. The national spending on defence has been cut by 450 per cent and most of this diverted to the welfare area, to pay for retirement pensions and superannuation payments. The average life expectancy is now 86 years for women and 80 for men.'*

Now: The basic tenets of this tongue-in-cheek prediction have been realised. Certainly there are magazines now devoted to the interests, finances and health issues of older people. The number of elderly men and women is increasing in all Western societies and the elderly proportion of the population is increasing progressively. There are many publications and magazines specifically for the elderly, and retirement homes and villages are proliferating. Many of the luxuries mentioned are becoming routine. Gero-power (called grey power at the moment) is now a political priority, and gero-spending is an issue for consumer marketeers.

Defence spending, unfortunately, remains high. Retirement and superannuation payments are huge and will become even bigger as the baby-boomers are starting to retire. Life expectancy is already about 83 in Japanese women and 80 in Japanese men but we are catching up.

Gero-power, whether it's called Grey power or Baby Boomer power, is here to stay.

Fifteen years from now: The trends that have occurred in the last 15 years have continued. Life expectancy in Japan is almost 88 in women and 85 in men. Facilities for the elderly (retirement villages, shopping centres, health facilities etc.) are continuing to expand and developers are focusing on these areas. A new industry of home-helpers has been developed, mostly part-timers in need of extra cash, who nevertheless have to meet strict criteria to become registered. Grans and grandpas have become among the biggest users of internet chat rooms, and explore the planet from their living rooms as they do things in cyberspace that they wish they had done when they were younger. Grans and grandpas have also become surrogate parents as they are the often part-time main grandkid-carers. Their kids (the parents of the grand-kids) are too busy making ends meet because they have to handle their large mortgages.

3. The death rate from coronary heart disease has fallen by a further 60 per cent to levels of the early 1900s before tobacco smoking became epidemic.'

Now: The death rate (at least for the middle-aged) has fallen by over

50 per cent to levels of the mid-1960s, when the curve for coronary deaths began to increase steeply. Levels in the 1900s were in fact very low and were similar to those of African and Asian countries before the industrial era. The number of heart attacks and strokes is actually increasing because of a larger proportion of the population living beyond the 70s and 80s (we've seen that clogging of the arteries is strongly age-related).

Fifteen years from now: The second part of this prediction has not been realised because of a triple whammy that has increased heart attacks and strokes in the community. I'm referring to the epidemic of obesity, metabolic syndrome and diabetes, all of which have aggravated clogging of the arteries. Their effects have combined with those of an ageing population. While total numbers of heart attacks and strokes have increased, medical treatment has made each attack less dangerous, so death rates per head of population have actually fallen. The load on hospital facilities has increased exponentially, with more procedures (angioplasties, stents, bypasses, implants, transplants etc.) being carried out at ever increasing cost to the community. The obligatory Medicare contribution for all workers has surged to 5 per cent of income.

4. *'Newborn babies have blood cholesterol levels measured from the same sample used to screen for the other inherited diseases of metabolism less common than familial hypercholesterolemia. Repeat samples are taken at six and twelve months for children who have blood cholesterol levels above the accepted upper limit, and dietary changes to reduce blood cholesterol levels are begun in those children over two years of age with persisting high blood cholesterol levels.'*

Now: This prediction was the result of my own research on inherited cholesterol in children and up to a point represented wishful thinking. Cord blood sampling has been found to be unreliable as a screening test for inherited high cholesterol because of a high rate of false positive and false negative diagnoses. Screening at age five days by measuring apoB in heel-prick blood has been more reliable, but is not yet practised routinely at any clinical centre. Children aged over two with familial hypercholesterolaemia are now treated routinely with a cholesterol-lowering diet.

Fifteen years from now: New methods of DNA analysis allow revival of heel-prick testing in children at the age of five days. A total genome scan reveals the genes that are likely to be involved in clogging of the arteries when the kids become adults. The activity of these genes is tested in other blood samples from the same child, as are factors that will determine the body's responsiveness to diet and drug treatment. A program, initially involving dietary modification but later in life drugs if necessary, is prescribed. Eventually, specific drugs will be prescribed for each individual in a specific dose that will inhibit the activity of the dangerous genes and promote protective genes. In this way, treatment is made doubly effective.

Evidence that treatment of children is effective in retarding or preventing clogging of the arteries in adults is being presented at international medical meetings. This will lead several years later to routine preventive measures being taken in children.

5. *'All children entering primary school have a coronary risk assessment performed. Their blood cholesterol / HDL ratio, blood pressure, obesity index and family history of coronary heart disease and other diseases are documented. Children with risk factors detected in the screening program are referred to appropriate clinics that advise the family regarding appropriate lifestyle changes. Risk factors are monitored regularly in children with one or more risk factors detected in the screening program.'*

Now: This prediction was also generated from my own research and preferences for 'what should be'. Risk factor assessment in childhood remains a black box and is only carried out at a few research centres around the world.

Fifteen years from now: It is recognised that the epidemic of obesity and diabetes, now affecting a large proportion of the population, has its roots in childhood. The previous black box has become a little greyer as health authorities examine and try to alter behaviour patterns in families. The measurement of gene activity and responses to diet and drugs (see no. 5 above) also helps.

'6. Children in primary school receive health education regarding the nature of coronary heart disease, its cause, and the role of the various risk factors in promoting coronary heart disease.'

Now: Education of children in the areas of lifestyle and risk factors is certainly happening. The learning curve is on the way up. Schools have started to take exercise and diet more seriously by looking at food choices in canteens and encouraging exercise both in and outside class times.

Fifteen years from now: Children receive even more detailed instruction on risk factors and risk behaviour related to smoking, alcohol, driving, relationships and nutrition. It's now 'cool' to eat low-chol lunches. Smoking is very 'uncool'.

7. *'Children attending high school have repeated coronary risk assessment performed, as above, and those with detectable risk factors again referred to specialist clinics for advice and monitoring.'*

Now: Not happening yet.

Fifteen years from now: Adolescent cardiovascular prevention clinics are established in routine practice, run by specialists and GPs and funded by a special government preventive health program. The whole family unit is involved, from kids to grans. Family intervention is the aim, with focus on the teenagers.

8. *'There is a national register for coronary heart and cardiovascular disease: all cases of angina, sudden death, heart attack and stroke are registered. A gradual and progressive decline in the incidence of all forms of coronary heart disease occurs.'*

Now: Part 1 of this prediction has occurred in certain research centres but not as a routine other than through death certificates. Part 2 has occurred for the middle-aged, but over the age of 65 numbers of cardiovascular events continue to increase because of ageing of the population and better medical care, so that an elderly person with an event is more likely to survive it and have a second later event.

Fifteen years from now: We've discussed trends of heart attack and stroke (see no. 3 above). This trend is likely to continue in the future, with an increase in the total numbers of heart attacks and strokes, but with each one being treated more effectively. Surviving one, two or even more cardiovascular episodes with little residual disability will occur quite commonly in the elderly.

9. *'A tablet for lowering blood cholesterol is available that is effective over a seven-day period, can be taken once weekly orally, has no side effects and has been shown to prevent the development of atherosclerosis.'*

Now: My first book was just before the statin era, and statins have almost fulfilled this prophecy although they are usually taken once daily. At this stage no drug has been available long enough, and treatment has generally not been started early enough and in sufficient dose, to prevent atherosclerosis. But it is a possible scenario. The issue of side effects remains but is less of a concern than in the pre-statin era. The latest treatment for high cholesterol—silencing RNA that turns off the gene for apoB synthesis—is now effective for more than seven days after a single injection, and is being trialled in humans.

Fifteen years from now. Gene silencing is a routine part of practice. A tiny implant is inserted under the skin and remains active for six months, so tablets or injections are no longer necessary. This technology is backed by genome-wide DNA scans that reveal the presence of genes that increase the risk of clogging of the arteries, as well as genes that promote unclogging. Genes that increase clogging are turned off by gene silencing. Gene amplification is a new technology that increases the activity of protective genes to promote unclogging. New methods are being developed that will enable gene activity to be modulated like dimmer switches for lights. The polypill has also been perfected as a result of several large studies with various combinations of medications. So doctors have a choice of effective preventive measures through a variety of medications. At present the polypill is the cheaper alternative, but DNA technology is becoming more cost-effective every year.

10. *'Patients with severe genetic high blood cholesterol levels (homozygous FH) are treated successfully by liver transplantation, which becomes a standard and safe technique. Those with single dose (heterozygous) FH are given a drug in a once-daily basis which stimulates LDL receptors in the liver and controls blood cholesterol levels.'*

Now: Both these predictions have been realised. Liver transplantation is routine for homozygous FH and statins are used routinely for heterozygous FH. ApoB silencing RNA is being trialled.

Fifteen years from now: The problems of transplant rejection have been overcome through the technologies of gene silencing and amplification. Cloning technology allows individuals to grow their own livers, kidneys, heart valves and blood vessels in the laboratory, providing a source for organ and tissue renewal when necessary. As an alternative to transplant, a battery-operated dialysis machine can be inserted into the abdominal cavity and continually filters LDL out of the blood.

References

Andersen KM, et al. 'Cholesterol and mortality: 30 years of follow-up from the Framingham study'. *JAMA* 1987; 257: 2176-80.

Austin MA, et al. 'Hypertriglyceridaemia as a cardiovascular risk factor'. *Am J Cardiol* 1998; 81: 7B-12B.

Baigent C, et al. 'Cholesterol Treatment Trialists. Efficacy and safety of cholesterol lowering treatment: prospective meta-analysis of data from 90,056 participants in 14 randomised trials of statins'. *Lancet* 2005; 366: 1267-78.

Brown MS, Goldstein JL. 'Receptor-mediated endocytosis: insights from the lipoprotein receptor system'. *Proc Natl Acad Sci USA* 1979; 76: 3330-7.

Ernst E, et al. *The desktop guide to complementary and alternative medicine: an evidence based approach*. Edinburgh: Mosby, 2001.

Frick MH, et al. 'Helsinki heart study: primary-prevention trial with gemfibrozil in middle-aged men with dyslipidemia'. *N Engl J Med* 1987; 317: 1237-45.

Gordon DJ, et al. 'High density lipoprotein cholesterol and cardiovascular disease: four prospective American studies'. *Circulation* 1989; 79: 8-15.

Hamilton-Craig I. *State of the Heart: Controlling Cholesterol and Triglycerides*. Barclay Sterling, 2007.

Hamilton-Craig I. 'MEDPED-FH. A new programme to improve the management of familial hypercholesterolaemia'. *Med J Aust* 1995;162:454-55.

Hamilton-Craig I. 'Statin-associated myopathy'. *Med J Aust* 2001;175:486-489.

Hamilton-Craig I. 'The Heart Protection Study- implications for clinical practice.' *Med J Aust* 2002;177:407-408.

Hamilton-Craig I. 'Case-finding for familial hypercholesterolaemia in the Asia-Pacific region'. *Sem Vasc Med* 2004;4:87-92.

Hunninghake DB. 'Therapeutic efficacy of the lipid-lowering armamentarium: the clinical benefits of aggressive lipid-lowering therapy'. *Am J Med* 1998; 104: 9S-13S.

Kannel WB. 'Metabolic risk factors for coronary heart disease in women: perspective from the Framingham study'. *Am Heart J* 1987; 114: 413-19.

Kavey RE, et al. 'American Heart Association guidelines for primary prevention of atherosclerotic cardiovascular disease beginning in childhood'. *Circulation* 2003; 107: 1562-66.

Lakka H-M, et al. 'The metabolic syndrome and total and cardiovascular disease mortality in middle-aged men'. *JAMA* 2002; 288: 2709-16.

Law MR, et al. 'By how much and how quickly does reduction in serum cholesterol concentration lower risk of ischaemic heart disease?' *Br Med J* 1994; 308: 367-73.

Mooney BD, et al. *Seafood The Good Food II*, 2002, CSIRO Marine Research.

'Multiple risk factor intervention trial. Risk factor changes and mortality results'. Multiple Risk Factor Intervention Trial Research Group. *JAMA* 1982; 248: 1465-77.

Nicholls SJ, et al. 'Statins, high-density lipoprotein cholesterol, and regression of coronary atherosclerosis'. *JAMA* 2007; 297: 499-508.

Ornish D, et al. 'Can lifestyle changes reverse coronary heart disease?' *Lancet* 1990;336:129-33.

Plaga BA. 'Treatment of childhood hypercholesterolemia with HMG-CoA reductase inhibitors'. *Ann Pharmacother* 1999; 33: 1224-7.

Fourth Euro. Soc. Task Force on Cardiovascular Disease Prevention in Clinical Practice, www.escardio.org, 2007.

Reaven G. 'Role of insulin resistance in human disease'. *Diabetes* 1988; 37: 1595-607.

Rodwell Williams, S. *Nutrition and Diet Therapy*, Times/Mosby College Publishing Co., 1985.

Ross R. 'Atherosclerosis—an inflammatory disease'. *N Engl J Med* 1999; 340: 115-26.

Roussouw JE, et al. 'The value of lowering cholesterol after myocardial infarction'. *N Engl J Med* 1990;323:1112-19.

Stein E (Ed), 'A symposium: rosuvastatin – an efficacy assessment based on pooled trial data', *Am J Cardiol* 2003; 91(suppl): 1C-27C.

Topol EJ. 'Intensive statin therapy—a sea change in cardiovascular prevention'. *New Engl J Med* 2004; 350: 1562-64.

Index

ACAT inhibitors 217–18
acute coronary syndrome (ACS)
  43
ageing see also elderly
  attitudes to 251–53
alcohol 120–25
  benefits 122
  excessive consumption
    121–22
  harmful effects 121–22
  recommendations 124–25
  red wine 122, 124, 125
  reducing intake 167
  SAFE Program 166–67
  standard drink 120–21
alpha-linolenic acid (ALA) 101
alternative therapies 112–19
American Heart Association 32,
  54
amlodipine 210
angina 22, 39, 40–41
angioplasty 238–40, 257
ankle-brachial blood pressure
  index 33
anorexia 80
aorta, clogging 20–21
aortic aneurysm 21
apo A-1 Milano 220
apoB 224
arcus senilis 82–83
arteries see also carotid arteries;
  coronary arteries
  clogging 16–22
  causes 26–30
  checking for 31–36
  illustration 17, 21
  inflammatory disease 27–28
  men versus women 245
  risk factors 19, 25
  symptoms 31
  seven step plan to clear 171–76
  unclogging 23–25, 237–42
arteriosclerosis 16
arthritis, effect of omega-3s 109
artichoke 114
aspirin 201–2, 209
atherosclerosis 16, 26
athrectomy 238
balloon angioplasty 238–40
behaviour change 168–70
beta-glucan 114
bile 80, 92
bile acid binding agents 216

blood fat levels
  acquired causes 78–81
  abnormal 72–73
  adults 71–73
  alcohol and 132
  children 73–75
  coffee and 128
  coronary risk factor 46
  high 77–87
  inherited 81–87
blood glucose disorders 141–46
blood homocysteine level 46–47
blood Lp(a) 46
blood pressure
  ankle-brachial blood pressure
    index 33
  coffee and 128
  high 47–48
  medication 198–203
  risk factor for heart attack and
    stroke 46
blood sampling procedure 89–90
breakfast 265–68
bypass surgery 241, 260
bypasses, natural 17, 39, 215
caffeine 127
calcification 18
calcium score, coronary 34–35
campestanol 218
campesterol 218
carbohydrates 130–34
cardiovascular death rates 153
cardiovascular disease
  benefits of treatment 55
  national register 297–98
  women versus men 244–47
carotid arteries 32, 238
carotid artery intima-medial
thickness (CIMT) 32
case studies
  Bill, heart attack 195–96
  Darren, alcohol-induced high
    blood cholesterol 123–24
  Jane, high triglycerides
    192–93
  John, exercise program 154
  John, thickened carotid arteries
    33
  Judith, low thyroid activity
    189–90
  Lyn, high blood HDL level
    154
  Mark, alcohol-induced high blood

cholesterol
  187–89
  Robert, high triglycerides
    190–92
  Stephen, familial
    hypercholesterolaemia 82–84
  Susan, diabetic 193–95
  Tim, heart attack risk 28–29
  Wayne, overfed, under-
    exercised, overweight
    182–87
cell membranes 59
cereals, carbohydrate content
  165–66
cerebral haemorrhage 20
cerebral infarction 19
cerebrovascular disease 19–20
CETP inhibitors 218–19
children
  blood fat levels 73–75
  cholesterol 73–75, 248
  coronary risk assessment
    296–97
  health education 297
  screening for cholesterol
    295–96
  unclogging arteries 248–50
chitosan 114–15
cholesterol 58–59
  absorption 92
  absorption inhibitors 216–17
  1in arterial walls 27
  balancing 91–95
  children 73–75
  dietary 92–95
  ester transfer protein inhibitors
    218–19
  esters 217
  foods containing 93–95
  genetic factors 93, 299
  HDL (good cholesterol)
    63–67
    effect of omega-3s 109
    functions 67
    heart attack rates with
      increasing levels 64
    measuring 68–69
    protective effects 65
    recommended levels 70, 179
  LDL (bad cholesterol) 68
    delivers cholesterol to
      arteries 27
    effect of omega-3s 109

heart attack rates with
increasing levels 64
measuring 68–69
receptors 68
recommended levels 70,
178–79
LDL/HDL imbalance 27
predictions for control 292–99
profiles, high/low risk 65–66
role 58
sources 91
testing your level 88–90
transport through body 59, 67
Cholesterol Club 233
cholesterol-lowering drugs 23–25,
216–19, 233–34, 298–99 *see
also* statins
cholestyramine 216
cigarette smoking 147–51
children 249
heart attacks and 148–49, 258
passive smoking 148
predictions 293
quitting 149, 151
risk factor for heart attack and
stroke 44, 46
clot-busters 240
clotting 29–30
clotting factors and triglycerides
225
cod liver oil 106, 110
coffee 126–29
colesavelam 216
Colestid 216
colestipol 216
collateral circulation 17, 39, 215
compliance 230–36
checklist 234
Minus-Factor 232–33, 235
@Plus-Factor 231, 234–35
studies 233
Support-Factor 236
cooking, low-cholesterol 261–64
coronary angiography 36, 260
coronary arteries 37–38
illustration 38
obstruction to blood flow
38–39
progression of clogging 17
symptoms of gradual
obstruction 39
symptoms of sudden
obstruction 39–42
coronary bypass 241
coronary calcium score (CCS)
34–35
coronary disease 19

national register 297–98
predictions 294–95
coronary risk factors 45–47, 51,
144, 160
C-reactive protein (CRP) 28, 47
CT coronary angiography 36
CT scans 34
cycling 158
death, sudden
result of exercise 156
result of heart attack 42
death rates
cardiovascular 153
link to overweight 136–37
desserts, recipes 289–91
diabetes 141–46
blood fats, rec. levels 179
blood glucose levels 78
risk factor for heart attack 47
diet
balanced 101–2
cholesterol lowering program
73
dietary traditions 98
fibre 131–32
low cholesterol cooking
261–64
double-blind study 113
drugs *see* medications
elderly
cholesterol control 254
cholesterol-lowering drugs
253–55
definition 252
predictions 293–94
unclogging arteries 251–55
endarterectomy 237–38
Eskimos' diet 106
essential fatty acids (EFAs) 100
ETC-216 220
evidence-based medicine 177
exercise, physical 152–60
benefits 153–54
body's response to 155–56
lack of, increases coronary
risk 46
program 156–59
SAFE Program 168
ezetimibe 210, 216
Ezetrol 216
familial combined hyperlipidaemia
(FCHL) 86
familial hypercholesterolaemia
(FH) 82–87
fat droplets 26–27

fats
controlling intake 102–4,
167–68
daily requirements 102
monounsaturated 61, 100
polyunsaturated 61, 100
saturated 61, 99
trans-saturated 101
fatty acids 60
monounsaturated 61, 100
polyunsaturated 61, 100
saturated 61, 99
femoral arteries 21
fenofibrate 226
fibrates 200, 226–27
fibre, dietary 131–32
fibrin 39
fibrinolytics 240
fish 106–11
dietary guidelines 110
mercury content 110
omega-3s in 108–9
fish oils 106
biological properties 227
capsules 109
for lowering triglycerides 227
precautions 110–11
protective effect 107
foam cells 27
foods
cholesterol-containing 93–95
suitable and less suitable
102–3
Framingham study 44, 55, 63,
127, 153
garlic 113–14
gemfibrozil 226
gene therapy 86
glucose 141–44, 164
glucose intolerance, impaired 78
glyceryl trinitrate (GTN) 40–41
glycogen 164
guar gum 114
HDL (good cholesterol) *see*
cholesterol
HDL-like proteins 220
health supplements 112–19
heart
abnormal rhythm 42
electrical instability 42
rapid heartbeat 257
surgery 241
heart attacks 37–43
age and gender of patients
41–42
cause 19
coffee and 127–28

fatality rates 45
measuring your risk 50–56
monitoring blood fats
following 259
pain 41–42
recovery 43
risk factors 44–49, 51, 144,
160
survival after 257–58
symptoms 41–42
unclogging arteries after
256–60
websites for estimating risk
54–55
women 245
heart muscle 40, 47
Heart Protection Study 246–47,
253–54
herbal supplements 112–19
homocysteine 46–47
homozygous FH 299
hormones, protective effects
245–46
hypoxia 40
immune system 80
impaired glucose tolerance 78
infarct 41
inflammatory markers 28
intestinal angina 22
intestines, clogging of arteries
22
Jezil 226
jogging 158
kidneys
clogging of arteries 22
kidney disease as risk factor 47
kidney failure 79–80
labels, food 102
LDL (bad cholesterol) see
cholesterol
LDL receptor activity 85
lecithin 116
legs, clogging of arteries 21–22
lifestyle program, cholesterol
lowering 173, 175
Lipidil 226
lipoprotein lipase 156
lipoproteins 59
liver
cholesterol source 91
function 68
transplantation 299
Lopid 226
lovastatin 206
magnetic resonance imaging
(MRI) 33–34
main courses, recipes 281–88

margarines, plant sterol 218
medications see also statins
ACAT inhibitors 217–18
bile acid binding agents 216
CETP inhibitors 218–19
cholesterol absorption
inhibitors 216–17
cholesterol-lowering 23–25,
72, 216–19, 233–34, 298–99
compliance 229–36
HDL-like proteins 220
influence on cholesterol 81
LDL-lowering drugs 23–24,
216–17, 234
PPAR alpha stimulants 219
side effects 230, 235
metabolic syndrome 141–46
mevinolin 206
monounsaturates, increasing intake
104
motivation 168–70
muscle aches 212
muscle melt-down 212–13
myocardial infarction 41
National Heart Foundation 54
nephrotic syndrome 79
New Zealand Cardiovascular Risk
Calculator 54–56, 172
nibbles, recipes 269–71
nicotine dependence 149–50
nicotinic acid 200–201, 227
oats 114
oestrogens 246
omega-3s 101
effects on arthritis and
inflammation 109
effects on LDL and HDL 109
effects on triglycerides 109
in fish 108–9
increasing intake 104
plant derived 109–10
protective effect 107
pactimibe 217–18
pain 40
palpitations, coffee and 128
pancreatitis, acute 166–67
patient, ideal 231
peroxisome proliferator activated
receptor 219
phospholipids 27
plant stanols 218
plant sterols 218
plaques
calcified 18
components 26–27
formation 18
illustration 17, 18

inflammatory cells 28
removing 237–38
rupture 25, 39
stabilising 25, 211–12
structure 18
unclogging 23–25
platelets 30
policosanol 115
polypill 210
polyunsaturates, increasing intake
104
PPAR alpha stimulants 219
pravastatin 253, 254
pregnancy 80
prescriptions 229, 231
progesterones 246
PROSPER Study 254
prostaglandins 107
psyllium 114
puddings, recipes 289–91
Questran 216
recipes
Apple crumble 291
Apples, baked 289
Baby spinach with water
chestnuts 288
Bananas 289
Beetroot salad 288
Butternut pumpkin shell 273
Carrot coriander soup 278
Cauliflower bisque 277
Cheat minestrone 279
Curried vegetable soup 280
Dried fruit compote 290
Dukkah 269
Dukkah-crumbed fish 283
Eggs 268
Fish chowder 278
Greek stuffed tomatoes 273
Hungarian paprika spread 271
Margo's new potato salad 288
Mousse 290
Muesli 267
Olive oil and balsamic vinegar
269
Pasta 285
Pastry cases 271
Poached salmon with mustard
dill sauce 283
Porridge 266
Potato and corn chowder 277
Rhubarb 290
Roast pumpkin and pea soup
276
Rocket and pear salad 287
Salade Nicoise 286
Smoked salmon 269

cutlets 281
Steak 281
Strudel 291
Stuffed capsicums 274
Stuffed mushrooms 275
Thai fish balls 284
Tomato and basil panzenella 287
Tuna pate 270
Turkey 282
Vegetable Pasties 275
Waldorf salad 288
Wasabi salmon 284
Yoghurt 268
regression 23
renal artery stenosis 22
resins 198–200
resting heart rate (RHR) 159
rhabdomyolysis 212–13
Richard, 7 step plan 171–76
risk assessment 50–56
risk factor 44
SAFE Program 162–70
salads, recipes 286–88
saturates, limiting intake 103–4
seafood, total fat, EPA, DHA and cholesterol in 108
Simons, Leon and Judy 233
simvastatin 217, 253
sitostanol 218
sitosterol 218
smoking see cigarette smoking
snacks 104, 269–71
soups, recipes 276–80
soy 115
stanols, plant 218
statins 204–14
  benefits 204–7, 208–9, 211, 221
  clinical trials 24–25, 207–8
  combination therapy 209–10
  for diabetics 145
  familial hypercholesterolaemia 84–85
  for lowering triglycerides 225
  side effects 212
  treatment with children 250
  treatment with elderly 253–55
  unclogging arteries 24–25, 204, 215
stenting 240, 257
sterols, plant 218
strokes 19–20
  cerebral haemorrhage 20
  cerebral infarction 19
  measuring your risk 50–56
  mini-stroke 20

risk factors 19, 44–49, 51
types 19–20
websites for estimating risk 54–55
sugars 131, 132, 133
  avoiding in SAFE Program 163–66
  foods containing 163, 165
supplements, health 112–19
surgery 237–42
  unclogging arteries after 256–60
swimming 158
tablet-taking 229–36
take-away foods 105
Task Force on Coronary Prevention 54
tendon xanthomas 82–83
testosterone 246
thrombosis 29–30
thrombus 29, 39
  dissolving 240
thyroid activity 79, 255
torcetrapib 218–19
transient ischaemic attack (TIA) 20
trans-saturated fats 101
  limiting intake 103–4
triglycerides 59–62, 222–28
  blood 61
  clogging of arteries 222–23
  and clotting factors 225
  drugs for controlling 225–27
  effect of omega-3s on 109
  energy source 60
  fatty acids 60–61
  functions 222
  glucose and 164
  high, inherited 86
  link with vascular disease 223–24
  in plaques 27
  recommended levels 179
  SAFE Program 162–70
troponin 42
vegetable dishes, recipes 272–75
vegetarians 117–18
ventricular fibrillation 42, 257
very low-density lipoproteins (VLDL) 68, 224
vitamin A 110
vitamin C 116
vitamin D 110
vitamin E 116–17
Vytorin 217
walking 157
wax alcohols 115

weight
  control 138–40
  gain 135–37, 141, 143, 149
  losing 138–40
  risk factor for heart attack and stroke 46
  weight for height chart 137
women
  cholesterol-lowering drugs 246
  heart attacks 245
  unclogging arteries 244–47
xanthelasmas 84
Zyban 151